DIFFERENTIAL

DIAGNOSIS

OF ARRHYTHMIAS

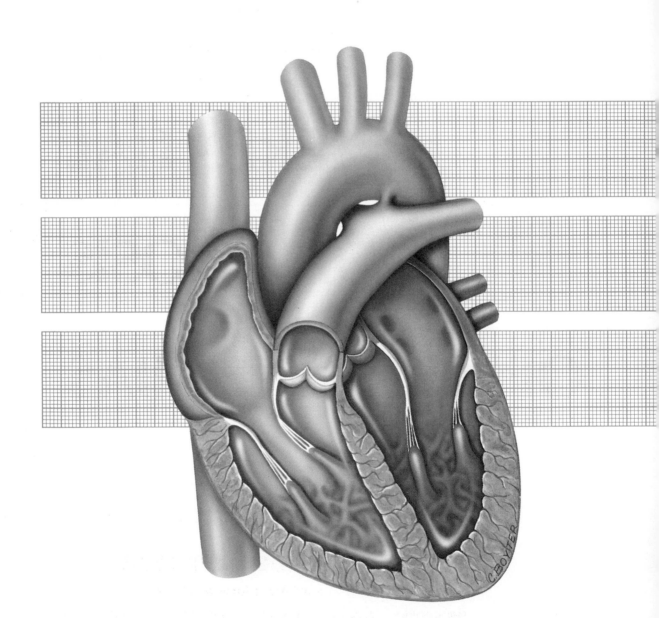

DALE DAVIS
RCT

General Partner
Cardiac Educational Resources
Mendham, New Jersey

DIFFERENTIAL

DIAGNOSIS

OF ARRHYTHMIAS

WB SAUNDERS COMPANY

Harcourt Brace Jovanovich, Inc.

PHILADELPHIA   LONDON   TORONTO   MONTREAL   SYDNEY   TOKYO

W. B. SAUNDERS COMPANY
Harcourt Brace Jovanovich, Inc.

The Curtis Center
Independence Square West
Philadelphia, PA 19106

Library of Congress Cataloging-in-Publication Data

Davis, Dale.
    Differential diagnosis of arrhythmias / Dale Davis.
        p.   cm.
    ISBN 0-7216-3691-8
    1. Arrhythmia—Diagnosis.   2. Diagnosis, Differential.   I. Title.
    [DNLM: 1. Arrhythmia—diagnosis.   2. Diagnosis, Differential.
    3. Electrocardiography—methods.   WG 330 D261d]
    RC685.A65D37   1991
    616.1'28—dc20
    DNLM/DLC
                                                    91-15027

Editor: Lisa A. Biello

DIFFERENTIAL DIAGNOSIS OF ARRHYTHMIAS   ISBN 0-7216-6708-2

Printed in the United States of America

Last digit is the print number: 9   8   7   6   5   4   3   2   1

PREFACE

Most students of arrhythmia have trouble with differential diagnosis, not only at the advanced level but also at the most basic level. And today students of arrhythmia interpretation are expected to perform at high levels of expertise and to be able to make accurate differential diagnoses.

This book devotes itself not only to learning the criteria for the arrhythmias, but also to acquiring the ability to differentiate them accurately from the other arrhythmias. I have taken the complex subject of arrhythmias and broken it down into manageable, simple learning steps, and yet still retained the integrity of the subject. I have chosen simplicity over exactness in some areas of the book to facilitate learning. Arrhythmia concepts are presented in a graduated series of isolated, step-by-step building blocks starting from the most basic and proceeding to the advanced. By following the same teaching format from chapter to chapter, a pattern of learning evolves. I feel that the simplistic approach to learning is best achieved by an extensive amount of illustrations, ECG examples, and practice strips.

Chapter one stresses the basic tenets of arrhythmia interpretation and is abundantly supplied with color illustrations. Chapters two through nine present each arrhythmia with a diagram of the electrical conduction system with the respective abnormality depicted, a criteria spreadsheet stressing differential diagnosis, and numerous ECG strips representing the abnormality. Differential diagnosis is discussed and illustrated in each chapter, allowing the student the opportunity to gain expertise with difficult arrhythmias. Dozens of practice strips with answers are found at the end of each chapter to allow the student to obtain necessary skills to become proficient in arrhythmia interpretation.

Chapter ten is solely devoted to differential diagnosis and correlates all the arrhythmias from the previous chapters, stressing the different approaches to accurate interpretation and giving clues to quick and accurate differential diagnosis.

This book is directed toward all students of arrhythmia who are interested in learning the basic and advanced arrhythmias and at the same time becoming proficient in differential diagnosis.

Acknowledgements

I want to thank my publisher, W.B. Saunders Company, for the latitude they permitted me in the book format and in the use of color illustrations. I'm indebted to my editor, Lisa Biello, who allowed me the freedom to develop my own ideas and who supported and guided me with her enthusiasm and expertise.

Many thanks to my designer, Patrick Turner, who turned my scribbles into masterpieces and who creatively developed the page by page layout for this manuscript.

And I'm grateful to the readers of my previous books whose suggestions and kind words guided me in the development of this publication.

CONTENTS

DIFFERENTIAL

DIAGNOSIS

OF ARRHYTHMIAS

1

THE BASICS

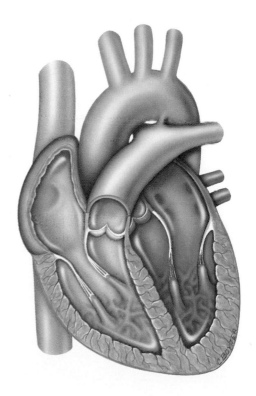

Anatomy

The heart is a muscular organ and is comprised of three layers. The outer layer is a serous membrane called the epicardium, the middle layer is cardiac muscle called the myocardium, and the inner layer is a serous membrane lining the inner surface and cavities of the heart called the endocardium.

The heart serves as a four-chambered pump for the blood flow throughout the body. It acts much like a filter in an aquarium, except on a grander scale. Just as dirty water flows into a receiving filter chamber, passes into a cleansing chamber for purification, and is then forced out again into the aquarium, the heart operates on the same principle, but with a four-chambered mechanism and instead of purification of fluid, oxygenation takes place.

The top two smaller chambers are called the left and right atria and are the receiving chambers. They are divided by the interatrial septum. The bottom two chambers are the left and right ventricles and they are the pumping chambers. They are divided by the thick interventricular septum.

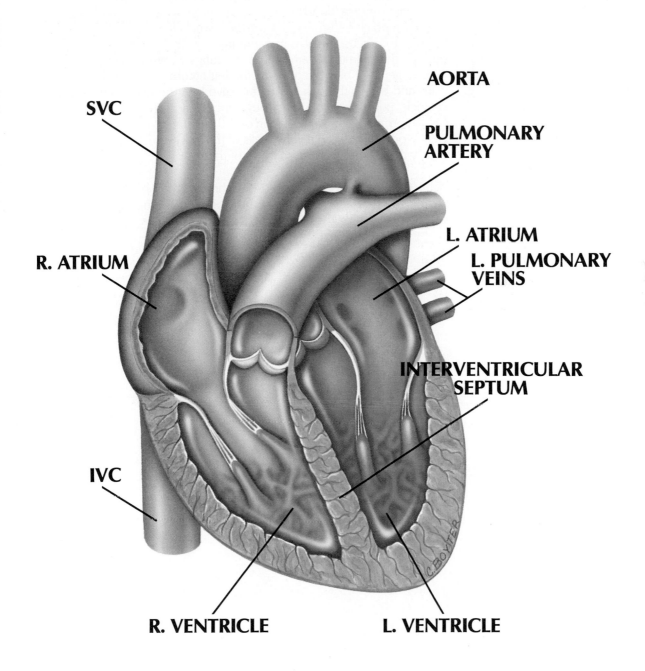

SVC

AORTA

PULMONARY
ARTERY

R. ATRIUM

L. ATRIUM

L. PULMONARY
VEINS

INTERVENTRICULAR
SEPTUM

IVC

R. VENTRICLE

L. VENTRICLE

C.BOYTER

Unoxygenated blood is received into the right atrium via the superior vena cava, which returns blood from the top portion of the body, and the inferior vena cava which returns blood from the lower half of the body. Blood flows through the tricuspid valve into the right ventricle and is then pumped through the pulmonary artery into the lungs where oxygenation occurs. The oxygenated blood returns to the left atrium via the four pulmonary veins and travels through the mitral valve into the left ventricle. The left ventricle pumps the blood through the aortic valve into the systemic circulation and allows oxygenation of all the tissues to occur. Because of the great work load placed on the walls of the left ventricle, they are approximately three times as thick as those of the right ventricle.

Although blood is constantly flowing through the heart's chambers, the heart muscle itself is not nourished by this flow and needs its own blood supply furnished by the left and right coronary arteries.

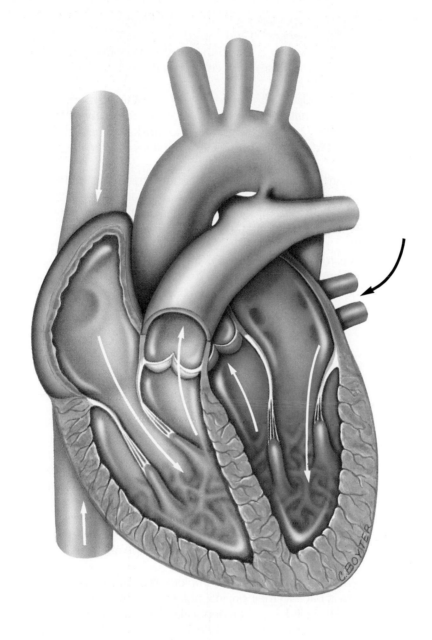

Electrophysiology

The heart maintains a rhythmic pumping action because of the electrical impulses generated and passed along the electrical wiring in the heart. This electrical wiring is called the electrical conduction system and transmits electrical impulses from cell to cell through the heart.

Each cardiac cell can begin and maintain rhythmic activity on its own. Certain anatomical areas display more automaticity than others. The sino-atrial (SA) node demonstrates the most automaticity in the heart and the atria, AV node, and ventricles exhibit less automaticity.

A cardiac cell is capable of responding to an electrical impulse passed along to it with an abrupt change in its electrical composition. Each cardiac cell is filled with and surrounded by electrical charges which change their polarity when they respond to electrical stimuli.

A cardiac cell transfers an electrical impulse to another cardiac cell with exceptional speed to make it appear as if all of the cells are responding at once to the electrical stimulus. Transmission velocity of electrical impulses vary from site to site within the heart:

AV node	200 mm/second
Ventricular muscle	400 mm/second
Atrial muscle	1000 mm/second
Purkinje system	4000 mm/second

When in the resting state, each cardiac cell is negatively charged on the inside of the cell membrane and positively charged on the outside of the cell membrane. Each cardiac cell is filled with and surrounded by a solution that contains ions. As a cardiac cell responds to an electrical stimulus it abruptly changes its respective polarity, by the movement of these ions inside and across the cell membrane, and the charges on the inside of the cell membrane systematically become positive from one end of the cell to the other, and those on the outside of the cell membrane become negative. This change in polarity is called depolarization.

When depolarization is complete, repolarization begins. All the charges revert back to their original polarity and the cycle is complete. Once the cardiac cells have been depolarized, another depolarization cannot occur until the first depolarization is completed. This is called the **absolute refractory period.** The **relative refractory period** follows immediately and occurs during repolarization, at which time the cardiac cells are capable of being depolarized but only by a strong stimulus.

The continuous depolarization and repolarization of all the cardiac cells is carried out by way of the electrical conduction system.

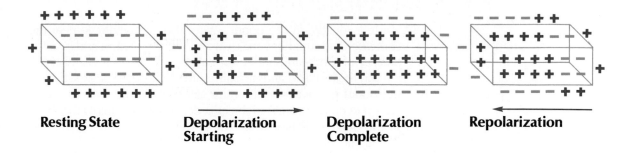

Resting State **Depolarization Starting** **Depolarization Complete** **Repolarization**

Electrical Conduction System

The ultimate goal of the conduction system is to transfer the electrical stimulation that begins in the SA node down to the ventricles. This is accomplished via the components of the electrical conduction system.

The **SA node** is located in the upper wall of the right ventricle near the junction between the superior vena cava and the right atrium and is called the pacemaker of the heart. Under normal circumstances it controls the heart's rate and rhythm. The sinus impulse spreads through the atria by way of the **internodal pathways** to the muscular walls of the atria and atrial depolarization occurs. The cells of the atria depolarize so rapidly that both atria appear to depolarize almost simultaneously, although the right atrium depolarizes slightly before the left atrium.

The depolarization wave travels to the **AV node** located on the right side of the interatrial septum on the floor of the right atrium and directly above the attachment of the tricuspid valve and is approximately one quarter of the size of the SA node. The depolarization wave, which has just depolarized both atria, delays at the AV node for approximately .10 second.

The **bundle of His** is a bundle of thin fibers on the right side of the interatrial septum and receives the depolarization wave after its delay at the AV node. It connects the AV node to the bundle branches.

The **right bundle branch** emerges from the bundle of His and transverses down the right side of the interventricular septum. It supplies the electrical impulses for the right ventricle.

The **left bundle branch** also arises from the bundle of His and immediately splits into two fascicles as it travels into the left ventricle. The **left anterior fascicle** provides the anterior and superior portions of the left ventricle with electrical impulses. The **left posterior fascicle** provides the posterior and inferior sections of the left ventricle with electrical impulses.

The right bundle branch and the left anterior and posterior fascicles divide into a network of fibers called the **Purkinje system**. These fibers terminate in the muscular walls of both the left and right ventricles and the electrical impulse is transmitted through them to the ventricular musculature and the ventricles depolarize.

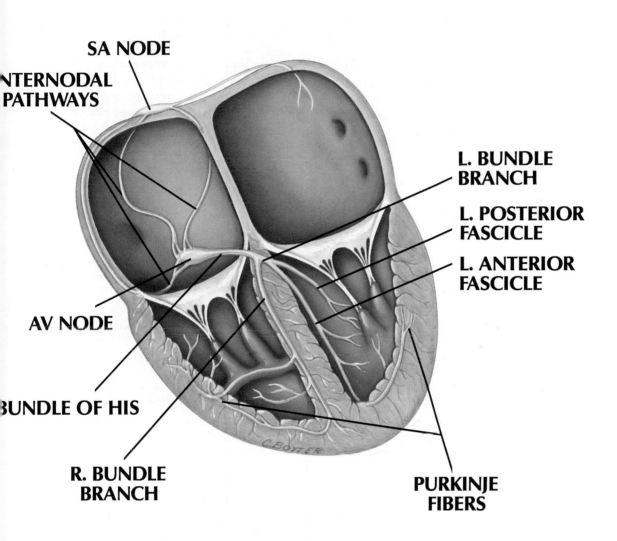

SA NODE

INTERNODAL PATHWAYS

L. BUNDLE BRANCH

L. POSTERIOR FASCICLE

L. ANTERIOR FASCICLE

AV NODE

BUNDLE OF HIS

R. BUNDLE BRANCH

PURKINJE FIBERS

C. BOYTER

Electrodes

Electrodes placed on the body pick up the electrical signals generated by the electrical conduction system and transmit them to ECG graph paper. Electrodes are placed on the four limbs and six designated areas on the chest and through various combinations of those electrodes, twelve different views of the same electrical activity are recorded and comprise a twelve lead ECG.

The three **standard leads** view the heart in the frontal plane and are composed of three pairs of electrodes—Lead I, Lead II, and Lead III. Each lead is composed of a negative and positive electrode and the ECG machine records the difference in electrical potential between them.

Lead I   Difference in electrical potential between the left arm and right arm.
Lead II   Difference in electrical potential between the left leg and right arm.
Lead III Difference in electrical potential between the left leg and left arm.

The standard leads are generally used for monitoring purposes and electrodes are placed on the four limbs or torso. Three electrodes give electrical information and the fourth electrode on the right leg merely stabilizes the tracing. This stabilizing electrode is called the ground electrode.

The three **augmented leads** aVR (augmented voltage of right arm), aVL (augmented voltage of left arm), and aVF (augmented voltage of left foot) also view the heart in the frontal plane and use the same three limbs, only in different combinations. These three leads record small deflections which are augmented by the ECG machine as signified by the small letter "a" in each of the leads.

Lead aVR   Right arm is the positive electrode compared to the left arm and left leg
Lead aVL   Left arm is the positive electrode compared to the right arm and the left leg
Lead aVF   Left foot is the positive electrode compared to the right arm and left arm

The six frontal or **precordial leads** view the heart in the horizontal plane.

Lead V1 and V2   are placed over the right ventricle
Lead V3 and V4   are placed over the interventricular septum
Lead V5 and V6   are placed over the left ventricle

12 LEAD ECG

STANDARD LEADS

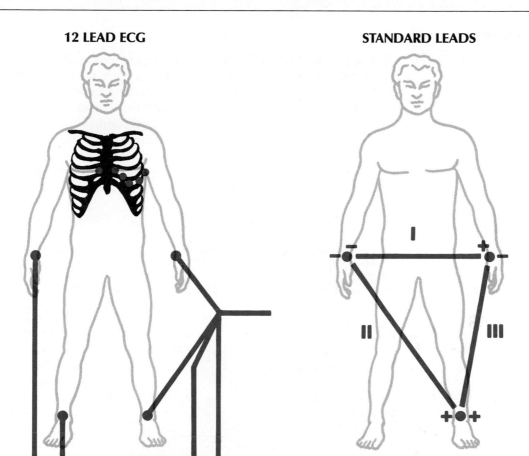

I

II

III

Precordial leads observe the heart in the horizontal plane

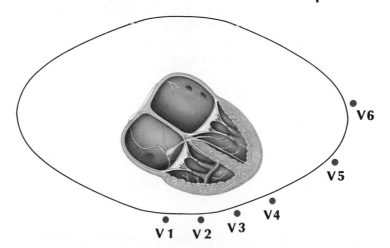

V6

V5

V4

V1 V2 V3

PQRST Waves and Intervals

Atrial and ventricular depolarization and repolarization are the electrical events that are recorded as waves on the ECG. SA node activity is not able to be recorded on an ECG. The SA node sends the depolarization wave out through the internodal pathways into the atrial musculature. The electrical impulse propagates from cell to cell instantly and the atria depolarize almost simultaneously. The average direction of depolarization is from the SA node outward and downward towards the patient's left side. The P wave represents atrial depolarization and is upright and slightly rounded.

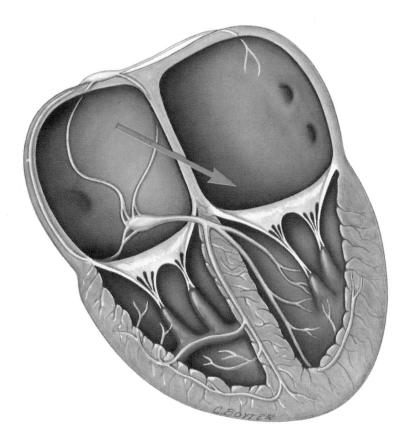

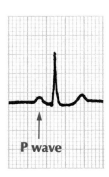

P wave

The atria repolarize and a **Ta** wave is recorded. This wave is usually not visible on an ECG because it correlates with ventricular depolarization.

The electrical impulse is transmitted to the AV node, bundle of His, bundle branches, into the Purkinje fibers in the ventricular musculature. The impulse propagates from cell to cell instantly and the ventricles depolarize almost simultaneously. The average direction of depolarization within the ventricles is downward and towards the patient's left side. A QRS complex is recorded which represents ventricular depolarization.

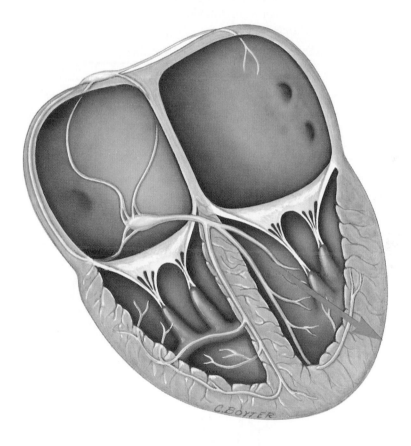

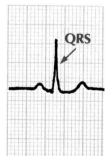

The QRS complex can be composed of a Q wave, R wave, and an S wave or any combination of waves. Various QRS configurations can be produced depending on lead placement and individuality. Each ventricular depolarization is called a QRS complex regardless of what waves make up the QRS.

Q wave is a <u>negative</u> wave preceding an R wave
R wave is a <u>positive</u> wave
S wave is a <u>negative</u> wave following an R wave

The negativity or positivity of a wave is based on its relationship to the baseline or the flat horizontal line recorded on the ECG paper called the **isoelectric line.**

DIFFERENT KINDS OF QRS COMPLEXES

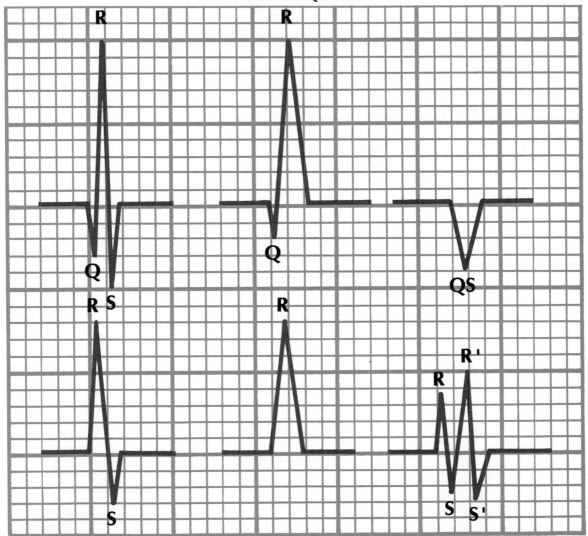

After the ventricles depolarize they must repolarize in order to regain their normal resting charge. Ventricular repolarization is represented on the ECG by a **T wave** which is normally upright, rounded, and larger than the P wave.

T WAVE

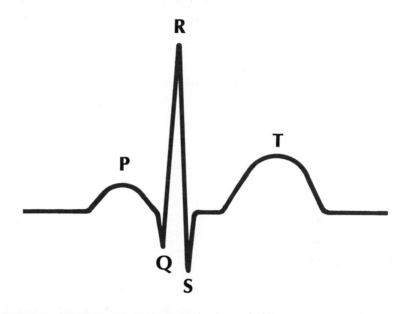

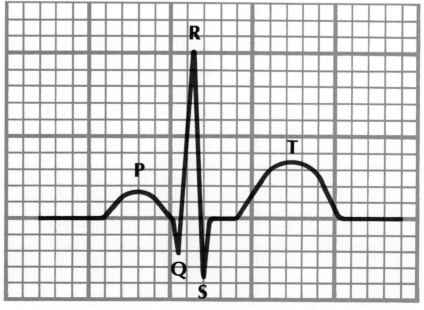

Once the PQRST waves are identified there are intervals and segments to be labeled and measured.

PR interval—The time from the beginning of the P wave up to the first wave of the QRS complex and represents the time from atrial depolarization up to but not including ventricular depolarization.

QRS interval—The time from the beginning of the first wave of the QRS complex until the last wave of the QRS complex and represents the time segment for ventricular depolarization.

ST segment—The time from the end of the last wave of the QRS complex until the beginning of the T wave and is a sensitive indicator of myocardial ischemia.

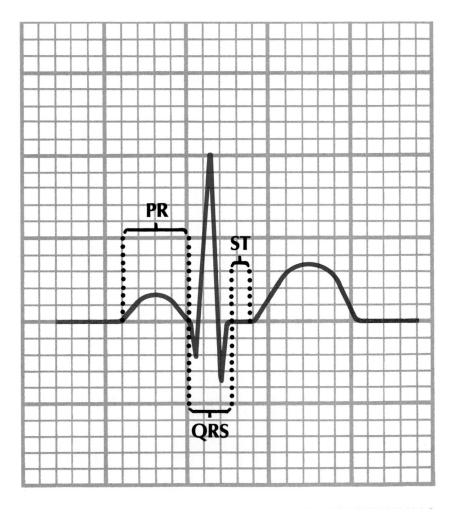

Now that you understand that the P wave represents atrial depolarization or electrical activity traveling through the conduction pathways of the atria and the QRS represents ventricular depolarization or electrical activity traveling through the conduction pathways in the ventricles it is logical to assume that if the electrical conduction is altered in any way within these chambers the P wave or the QRS will be changed also.

Measurements

The ECG is recorded on standardized graph paper. Voltage is measured vertically as the paper is divided into 1 mm divisions by the small, light lines and 5 mm divisions by the large, dark lines.

Q waves are measured to determine if they are diagnostic of infarction. R waves and S waves are measured to determine if they meet the voltage criteria for hypertrophy. R wave voltages are compared to previous ECGs for loss of R wave height which could be indicative of infarction or simply an inadvertent change in electrode position.

The ST segment is examined to ensure that it is neither more than 1mm above or below the baseline or isoelectric line on the ECG.

VOLTAGE

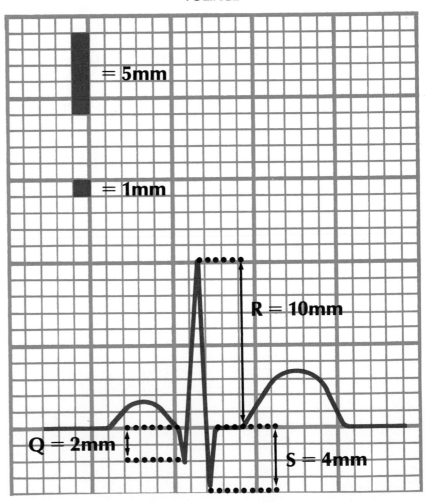

Time is measured horizontally as the paper is divided into .04 second divisions by the small, light lines and .20 second by the large, dark lines. The PR interval is measured from the beginning of the P wave to the first wave of the QRS complex. The normal PR interval is .12-.20 second. Anything shorter than .12 second constitutes accelerated AV conduction and indicates rapid conduction from the atria to the ventricles usually by way of an accessory conduction pathway that bypasses the AV node and therefore shortens conduction time.

A PR interval longer than .20 second constitutes first degree AV block and indicates a slowing of conduction from the atria to the ventricles.

TIME

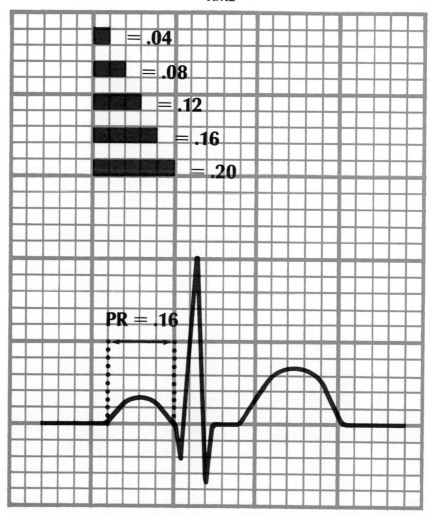

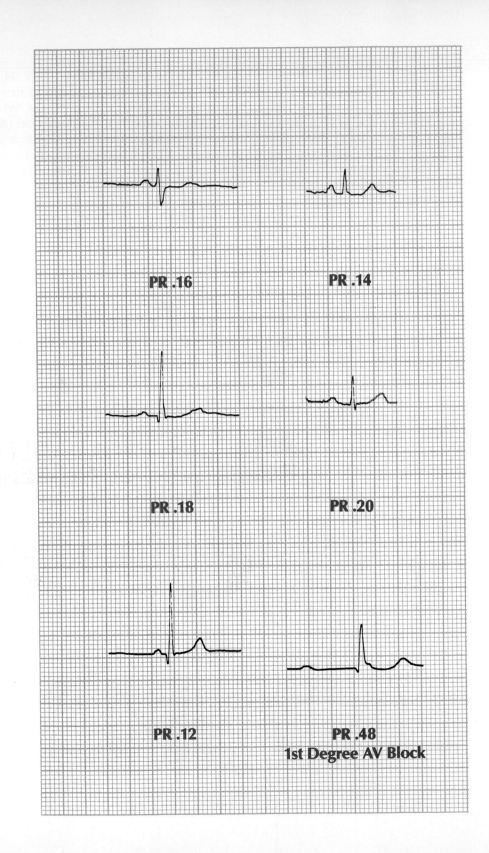

PR .16

PR .14

PR .18

PR .20

PR .12

PR .48
1st Degree AV Block

The QRS interval is measured from the beginning of the first wave of the QRS complex to the end of the last wave of the QRS complex. The normal QRS interval measures .04-.11 second. Anything longer than .11 second constitutes bundle branch block and represents a slowing of conduction through abnormal conduction pathways in the ventricles because of the blockage of one of the bundle branches.

If the right bundle branch is impaired, electrical depolarization will travel down the left bundle branch and proceed with depolarization and then through slower connection pathways in the ventricular muscle depolarize the right ventricle. This slowness of conduction gives rise to the widened QRS complex.

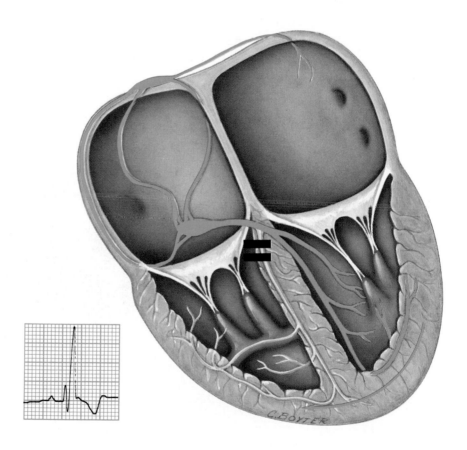

If the main left bundle branch is impaired electrical depolarization will proceed down the right bundle branch and cause right ventricular depolarization and then through slower conduction pathways in the ventricular muscle depolarize the left ventricle. This slowness of conduction gives rise to the widened QRS complex.

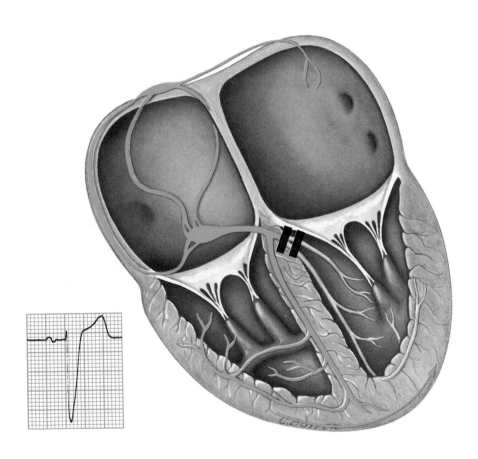

DIFFERENTIAL DIAGNOSIS OF ARRHYTHMIAS

In bundle branch block conduction is normal above the bundle branches so the P wave and PR interval will be normal. Only the QRS complex will be widened to .12 second or greater because of the delay in conduction through abnormal conduction pathways.

TIME

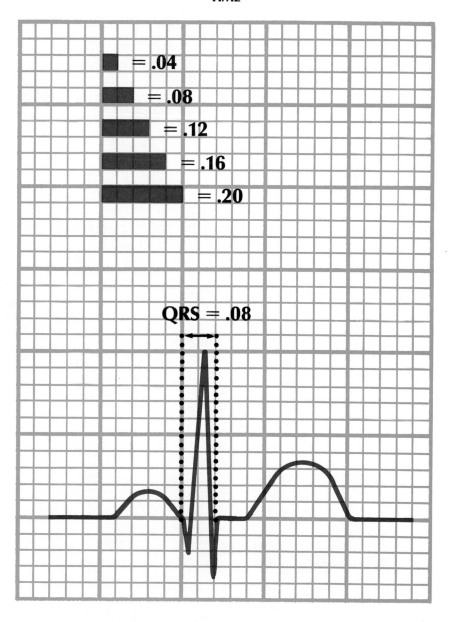

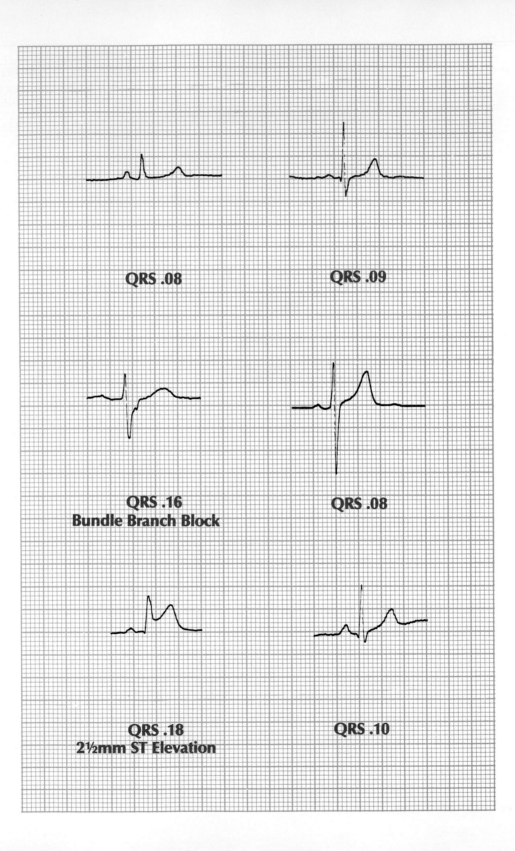

QRS .08

QRS .09

QRS .16
Bundle Branch Block

QRS .08

QRS .18
2½mm ST Elevation

QRS .10

Heart Rate

The heart rate can be calculated numerous ways but I've found the 300-150-100 method to be the best. It's quick, easy, and accurate and doesn't require the use of rate rulers or calculations.

Utilizing and memorizing the numbers **300-150-100-75-60-50-43** you can calculate the heart rate by finding an R wave that falls on or near a heavy black line on the ECG paper. Count the heavy black lines to the right of the R wave until the next R wave is recorded. Count these lines using the seven memorized numbers. The first line to the right is the 300 line, the second line is the 150 line, the third line is the 100 line, the fourth line is the 75 line, and so forth. If the next R wave lands on the fourth or 75 line, the heart rate is 75 beats per minute.

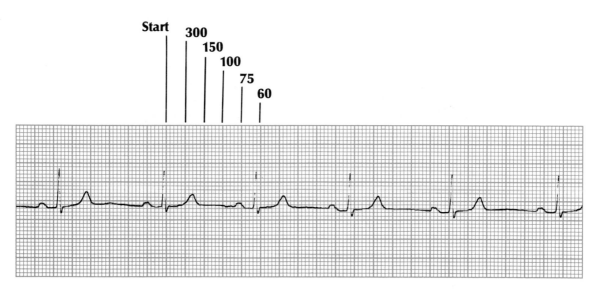

The heart rate is slightly faster than 60 beats per minute.

Heart Rhythms

The SA node is the pacemaker of the heart and rhythms beginning in the SA node are called sinus rhythms. In sinus rhythm the P waves and QRS complexes should resemble each other and the PR interval should remain the same throughout the tracing. The **P to P interval** (distance from P wave to P wave) and the **R to R interval** (distance from R wave to R wave) should be the same.

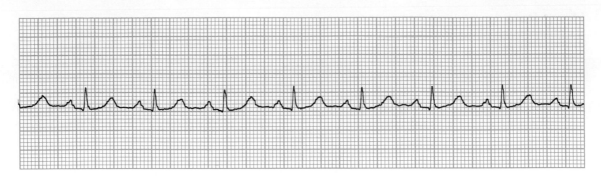

The heart rate is approximately 80 beats per minute.

If the sinus rate is below 60 beats per minute the rhythm is called **sinus bradycardia.** This slower rate is common when resting and in trained athletes. Sinus rates between 60-100 beats per minute are in the most common range and are called **sinus rhythm.** Sinus rates above 100 beats per minute are called **sinus tachycardia** and occur normally when exercising. These rhythms should have P-P and R-R cycles that are regular and PR intervals which do not vary throughout the ECG.

Each of these rhythms is normal if it occurs at an appropriate time. A sinus tachycardia occurring during rest would be inappropriate as would a sinus bradycardia while running on a treadmill.

Sinus arrhythmia is a rhythm beginning in the sinus node where the P-P and R-R cycles vary more than .16 second and this variation often coincides with respiration. R-R and P-P cycles gradually lengthen during inspiration and shorten during expiration. Sinus arrhythmia usually occurs during slow sinus rates or frequently in children.

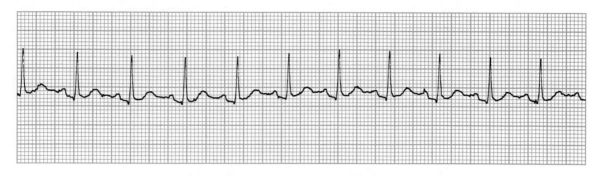

The heart rate is slightly faster than 100 beats per minute.

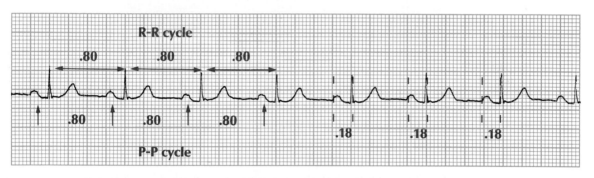

**Both the P-P and R-R cycle measure .80 second throughout the tracing
and the PR interval is constant at .18 second.**

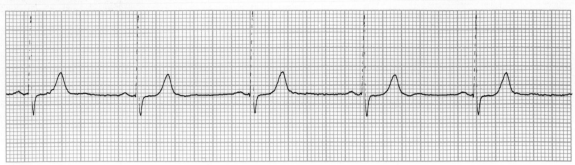

Sinus Bradycardia 51 beats per minute

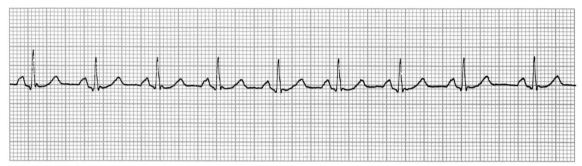

Sinus Rhythm 94 beats per minute

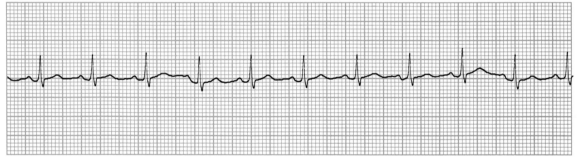

Sinus Tachycardia 110 beats per minute

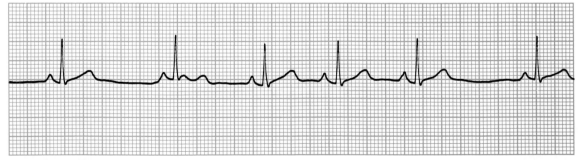

Sinus Arrhythmia

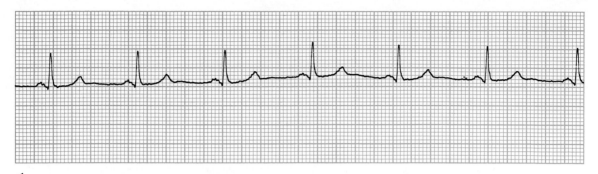

1   **PR =**   **QRS =**   **Rate =**   **Rhythm =**

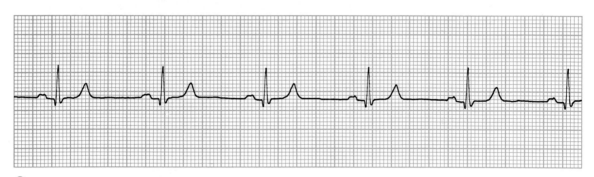

2   **PR =**   **QRS =**   **Rate =**   **Rhythm =**

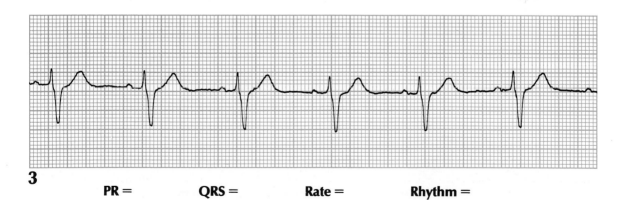

3   **PR =**   **QRS =**   **Rate =**   **Rhythm =**

PRACTICE ECGs

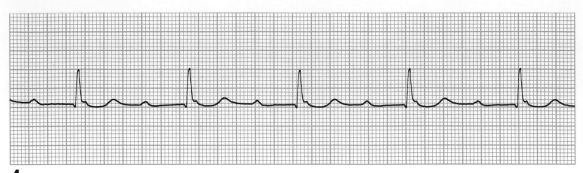

4
       PR =   **QRS =**   **Rate =**   **Rhythm =**

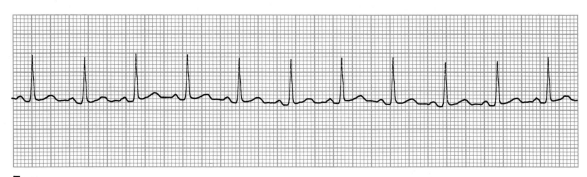

5
       PR =   **QRS =**   **Rate =**   **Rhythm =**

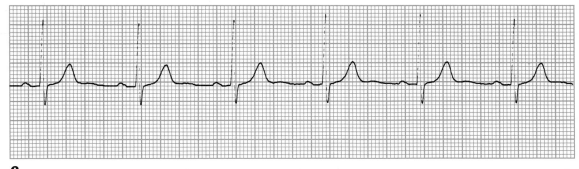

6
       PR =   **QRS =**   **Rate =**   **Rhythm =**

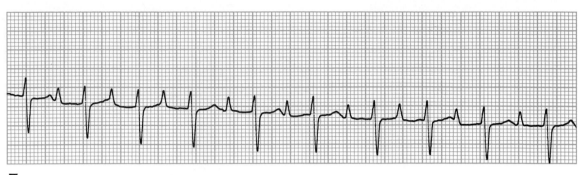

7   PR =   QRS =   Rate =   Rhythm =

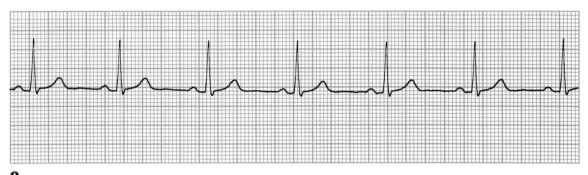

8   PR =   QRS =   Rate =   Rhythm =

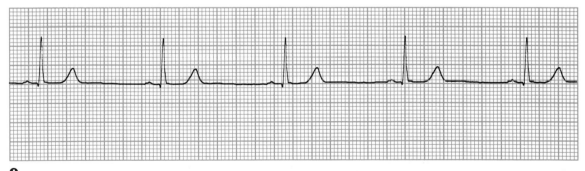

9   PR =   QRS =   Rate =   Rhythm =

PRACTICE ECGs

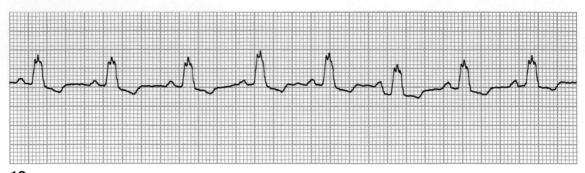

10
        PR =   **QRS =**   **Rate =**   **Rhythm =**

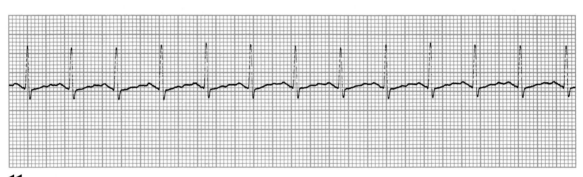

11
        PR =   **QRS =**   **Rate =**   **Rhythm =**

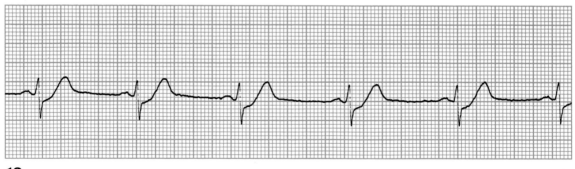

12
        PR =   **QRS =**   **Rate =**   **Rhythm =**

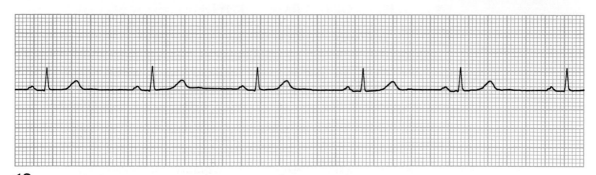

13   PR =   QRS =   Rate =   Rhythm =

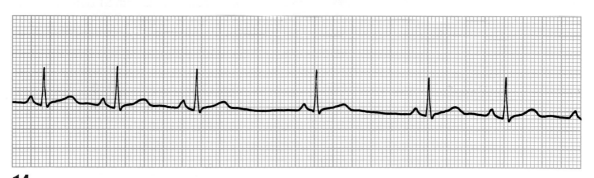

14   PR =   QRS =   Rate =   Rhythm =

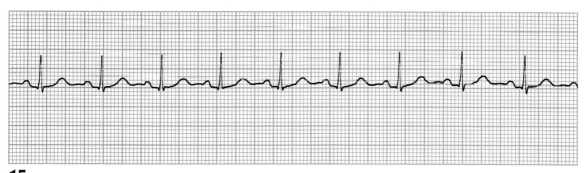

15   PR =   QRS =   Rate =   Rhythm =

Answers To Practice ECGs

	PR	QRS	RATE	RHYTHM
1.	.12	.08	65	Normal sinus rhythm
2.	.18	.10	55	Sinus bradycardia
3.	.16	.14	62	Sinus rhythm with bundle branch block
4.	.48	.16	50	Sinus bradycardia with bundle branch block and first degree AV block
5.	.14	.08	100	Sinus rhythm
6.	.20	.08	58	Sinus bradycardia
7.	.28	.08	94	Sinus rhythm with first degree AV block
8.	.18	.10	66	Sinus rhythm
9.	.16	.08	47	Sinus bradycardia
10.	.16	.14	80	Sinus rhythm with bundle branch block
11.	.14	.08	125	Sinus tachycardia
12.	.16	.08	55	Sinus bradycardia with ST depression
13.	.16	.06	54	Sinus bradycardia
14.	.16	.06	60	Sinus arrhythmia
15.	.16	.08	94	Sinus rhythm

DIFFERENTIAL DIAGNOSIS OF ARRHYTHMIAS

INTRODUCING ARRHYTHMIAS AND INTERPRETATION

Enhanced Automaticity—Premature Beats

Unifocal versus Multifocal

Compensatory versus Noncompensatory Pause

Escape Beats

Interpretation

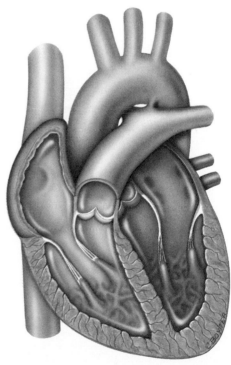

Enhanced Automaticity—Premature Beats

Cardiac cells possess the electrophysiological property of automaticity. The sinus node possesses automatic cells with the highest degree of automaticity with an inherent rate of approximately 60-100 impulses per minute and therefore becomes the pacemaker of the heart. The AV node's inherent rate is approximately 40-60 per minute and the ventricles possess an inherent rate of 40 or less impulses per minute. If areas or **foci** in the atria, around the AV junction where the atrial fibers enter the AV node and the area in which the AV node extends into the bundle of His, or in the ventricles, temporarily increase automaticity, they too can initiate an electrical impulse, overriding the SA node and produce an extra, early beat called an **extrasystole, ectopic beat, premature beat** or **premature contraction.** These premature beats interrupt the regular dominant sinus rhythm of the heart by arriving early and are named according to the area of the heart they originate in.

ATRIAL PREMATURE CONTRACTION

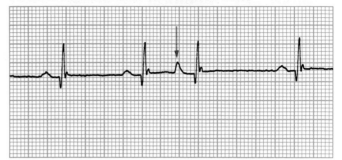

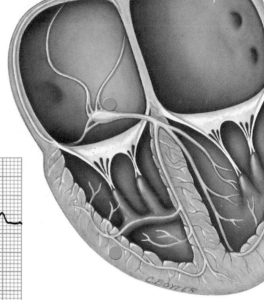

JUNCTIONAL PREMATURE CONTRACTION

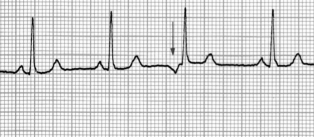

VENTRICULAR PREMATURE CONTRACTION

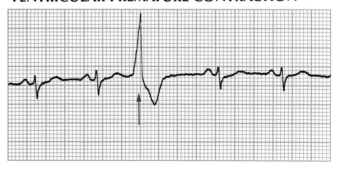

Unifocal and Multifocal

If only one area or focus in either the atria, AV junction, or ventricles fires, then the term used for these premature contractions is **unifocal** (one focus). If more than one focus in either the atria, AV junction, or ventricles fires, then the premature beats are considered **multifocal** (more than one focus).

To differentiate between unifocal and multifocal **atrial premature contractions (APCs)** one must look to the P wave. The P wave represents atrial depolarization and normal depolarization occurs from the SA node outward and downward. This normal atrial depolarization produces an upright, rounded P wave. If the APC originates from a focus in the opposite atrium, then depolarization of the atria will occur from a different direction and the P wave will have a different configuration. Unifocal APCs will all have an ectopic P wave bearing the same configuration. Multifocal APCs will display P waves of various shapes and forms.

To differentiate between unifocal and multifocal **AV junctional premature contractions (JPCs)** one again must look to the P wave. With JPCs the P wave will be inverted because the atria are depolarized from the AV junction backwards to the atria recording a backwards P wave. If the JPCs are unifocal, all the inverted P waves will be similar. If the JPCs are multifocal, the inverted P waves will have various shapes and forms.

To differentiate between unifocal and multifocal **ventricular premature contractions (VPCs)** one has to look at the QRS complexes. A VPC is initiated in a focus in one ventricle. The ventricle depolarizes and then with delay, through abnormal conduction pathways in the ventricular myocardium, depolarizes the other ventricle. The delay and change in direction of conduction causes a widened and bizarre looking QRS complex. Unifocal VPCs look alike and multifocal VPCs have various configurations.

UNIFOCAL APCs

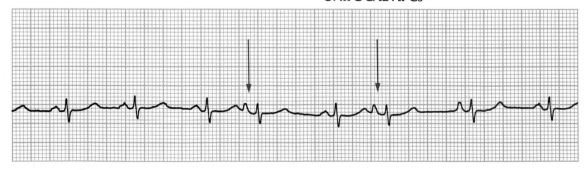

DIFFERENTIAL DIAGNOSIS OF ARRHYTHMIAS

MULTIFOCAL APCs

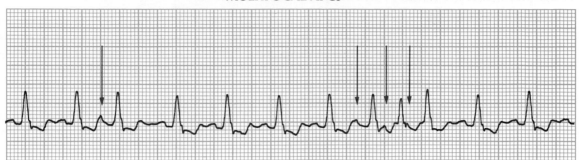

UNIFOCAL VPCs

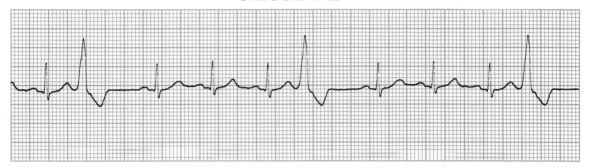

MULTIFOCAL VPCs

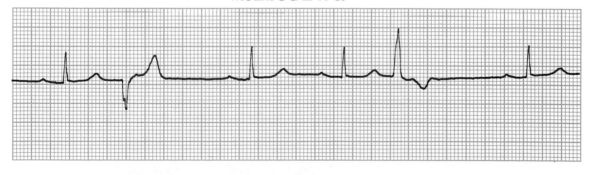

Compensatory Versus Noncompensatory Pauses

APCs, JPCs, and VPCs are all premature beats, that is they interrupt the rate of the regular cardiac rhythm by arriving earlier than expected. A ventricular pause normally follows premature beats to allow the cells of the heart time to return to their normal resting state and prepare for the next cycle.

A VPC is usually followed by a compensatory pause. The VPC arises from a focus in the ventricles and does not disrupt the rhythm of the SA node because it does not depolarize it. The sinus cycle is not disturbed by the VPC and after the ventricular pause continues on when expected. The R-R interval containing the premature beat is two times the R-R interval of the basic rhythm.

An APC or JPC is usually followed by a noncompensatory pause. The sinus node is depolarized by the premature beat and its regularity is disturbed and the sinus beat following the pause occurs sooner than expected.

COMPENSATORY PAUSE

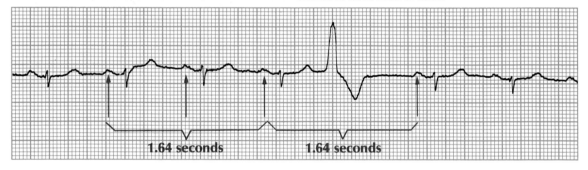

1.64 seconds 1.64 seconds

P wave cycle remains regular.

NONCOMPENSATORY PAUSE

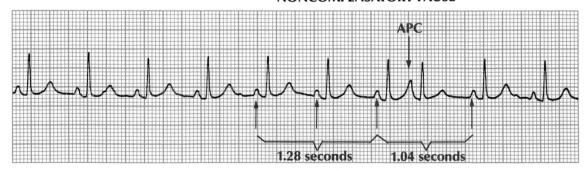

APC

1.28 seconds 1.04 seconds

P wave cycle is disrupted and sinus P wave following APC arrives sooner than expected.

A premature beat is attached to the previous beat by a set distance called a coupling interval. Unifocal premature beats display a constant coupling interval while multi-focal premature beats exhibit a varying coupling interval. Normally, a premature beat has a constant coupling interval because the impulse formation of the ectopic focus is dependent upon the preceding beat of the basic rhythm.

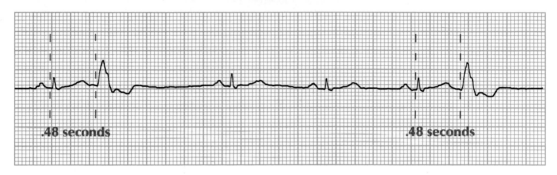

Unifocal VPCs displaying a constant coupling interval.

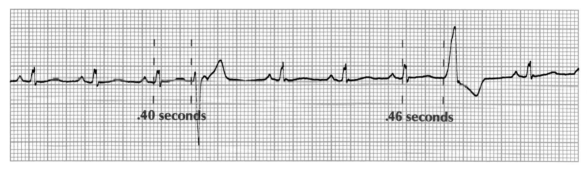

Multifocal VPCs demonstrating varying coupling interval.

Escape Beats

Opposite to enhanced automaticity is the SA node's slowing, cessation, or slow response following an ectopic beat, alerting a focus around the AV junction or in the ventricles to issue an escape beat. Escape beats save the heart from long ventricular pauses or asystole. Junctional escape beats are late in relation to the dominant cardiac rhythm and are either preceded by or followed by inverted, ectopic P waves or display no ectopic P wave and have a QRS that resembles that of the regular cardiac rhythm. Ventricular escape beats are late in relation to the dominant cardiac rhythm, have no associated ectopic P waves and display a wide and bizarre QRS complex. Escape beats occur isolated, in pairs, or in runs. Escape beats are attached to the previous beat by a distance called an **escape interval.** Escape beats arising from the same focus display a constant escape interval.

Junctional escape beat

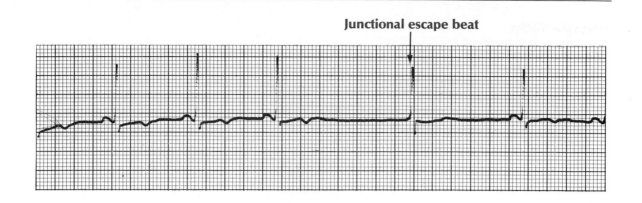

Ventricular escape beat

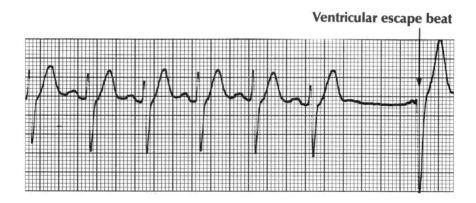

ESCAPE INTERVAL

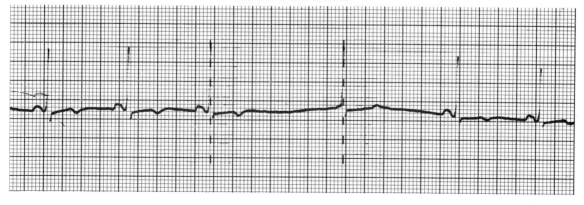

Interpretation

Arrhythmia interpretation requires a logical order of interpretive steps in order to be successful. I'm going to relate an interpretive pattern for arrhythmias that I use and works well for me:

1. Scan the entire strip to get an overall impression and check for regularity of rhythm.
2. Identify P waves, PR intervals, QRS complexes, ST segments and T waves.
3. Measure P-P and R-R cycles to ascertain regularity.
4. Measure PR and QRS intervals.
5. Calculate rate and rhythm.
6. Start at the beginning of the strip and identify each beat and pause that occurs and verify that the final interpretation meets all necessary criteria.

3

APCS, JPCS, AND VPCS

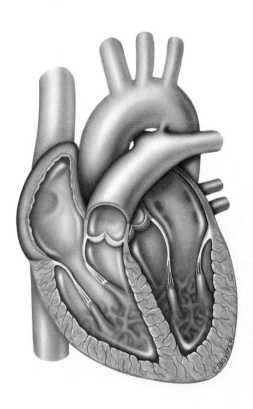

APC JPC VPC

APC

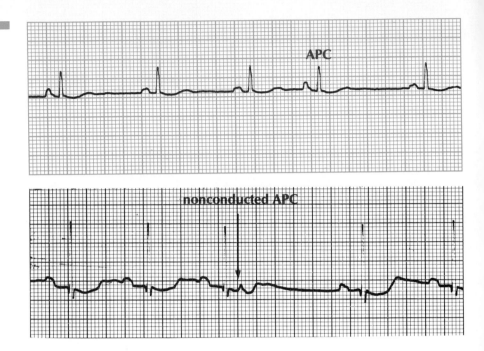

APC

nonconducted APC

CRITERIA

1. Early, different looking upright P wave followed by a QRS resembling the QRS of the dominant rhythm.

2. Noncompensatory pause following the APC.

3. If an ectopic P wave arrives extremely early, it may be unable to conduct to the ventricles (nonconducted APC) and will not be followed by a QRS complex.

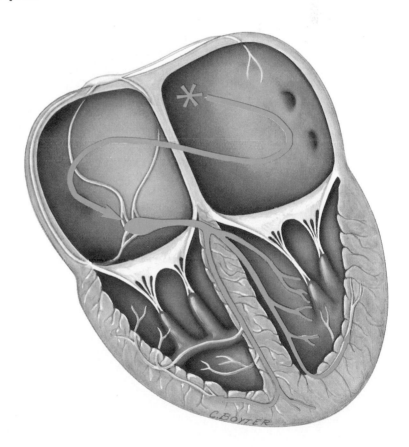

APC JPC VPC

JPC

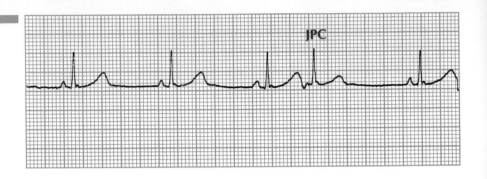

CRITERIA

1. **Early QRS resembling QRS of dominant rhythm with no visible P wave, or an inverted P wave preceding or following QRS.**

2. **Noncompensatory pause following the JPC.**

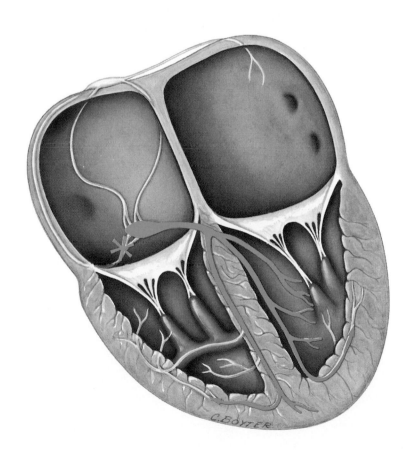

APC JPC VPC

VPC

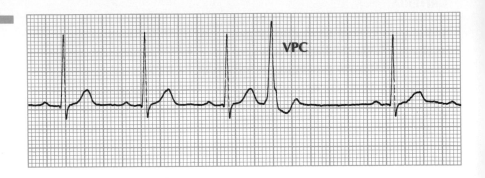

CRITERIA

1. **Early, wide and bizarre (.12 second or greater) QRS complex**

2. **Compensatory pause following VPC**

3. **No ectopic P wave**

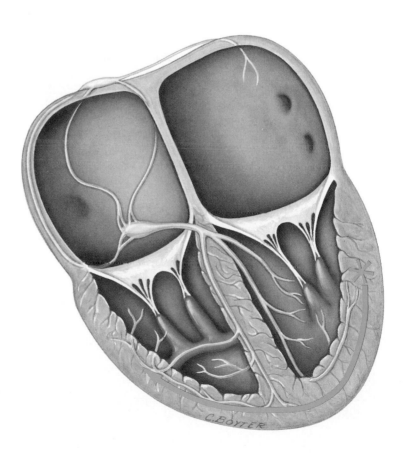

APCs, JPCs, and VPCs are all premature beats, that is they interrupt the regular rate of the dominant rhythm of the heart by arriving earlier than expected. Premature beats can be isolated events, occur every other beat (**bigeminy**), every third beat (**trigeminy**), every fourth beat (**quadrigeminy**), in pairs, or as runs of premature beats.

APCs

An APC is a premature beat, initiated in one area of the atria other than the SA node. This causes the atria to depolarize in a different direction than normal giving rise to a P wave different in configuration than the sinus P wave. Commonly, the early P wave is hidden in the previous T wave and deforms its shape. Conduction to the ventricles follows through normal conduction pathways, recording a QRS with the same configuration as the sinus rhythm and a ventricular pause following it. The SA node's cycle is disturbed as it is depolarized by the premature contraction causing it to reset itself and arrive earlier than expected, giving rise to a noncompensatory pause following the APC.

Hidden ectopic P wave

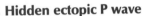

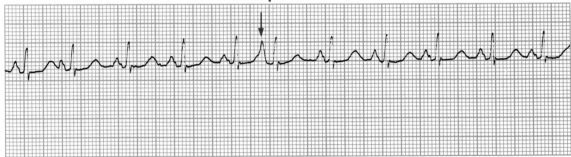

Sinus tachycardia with one isolated APC.

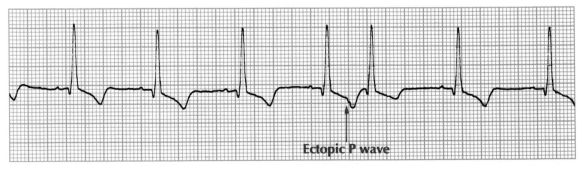

Ectopic P wave

Sinus rhythm with one isolated APC.

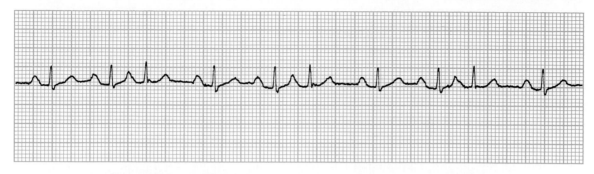

Sinus rhythm with first degree AV block with APCs in trigeminy.

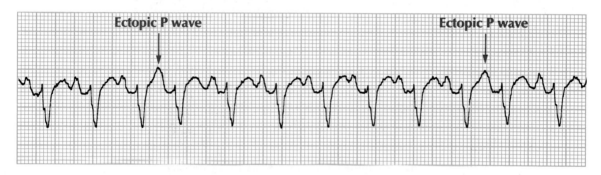

Ectopic P wave

Ectopic P wave

Sinus tachycardia with bundle branch block and two isolated APCs.

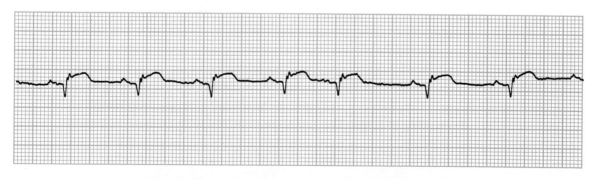

Sinus rhythm with ST elevation and one isolated APC.

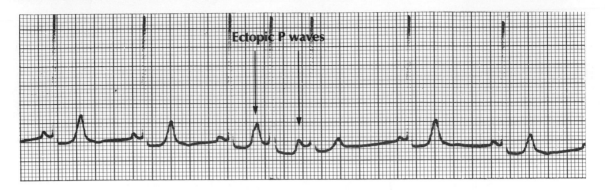

Sinus rhythm with a pair of APCs.

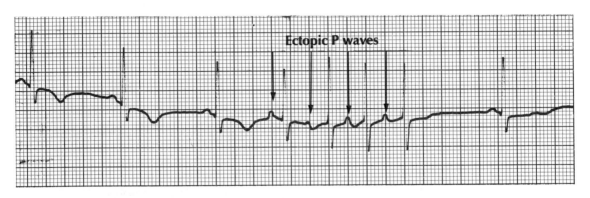

Sinus rhythm with four APCs in a row.

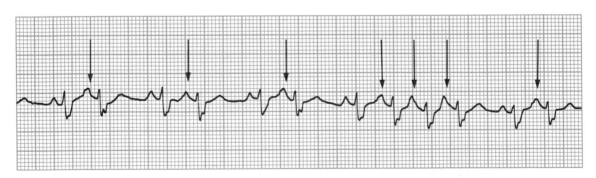

Sinus rhythm with four isolated APCs in bigeminy and one episode of three APCs in a row. The APCs are depicted with arrows.

DIFFERENTIAL DIAGNOSIS OF ARRHYTHMIAS

If an APC arrives very prematurely it may find the AV node still busy or refractory from the previous sinus beat and unable to conduct the APCs electrical impulse down to the ventricles to produce a QRS. An early, ectopic P wave will be recorded with a ventricular pause following it and no QRS complex. This is termed a nonconducted APC and is the most common cause of a ventricular pause. Always check the T wave before a ventricular pause for hidden ectopic P waves. It is important to properly identify the cause of ventricular pauses and rule out more dangerous arrhythmias.

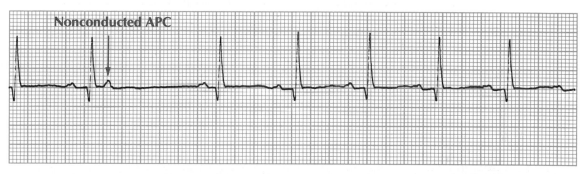

Sinus rhythm with first degree AV block and one nonconducted APC.

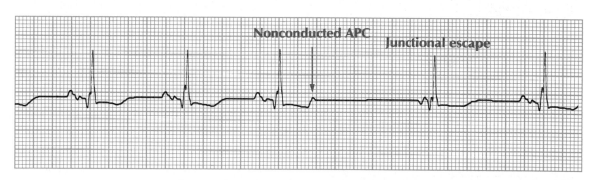

Sinus rhythm with one nonconducted APC followed by a junctional escape beat.

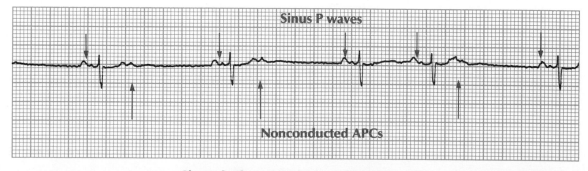

Sinus rhythm at 79 beats per minute with nonconducted APCs in bigeminy.

JPCs

A JPC is a premature beat initiated in an area around the AV junction. It depolarizes the atria in a backward or retrograde fashion as depolarization proceeds from the AV junction back to the atria, producing a backwards or inverted premature P wave. Conduction also travels downward to the ventricles through normal conduction pathways producing a QRS complex with the same configuration as the dominant rhythm and a ventricular pause following it. The SA node's cycle is disturbed as it is depolarized by the premature contraction causing it to reset itself and arrive earlier than expected, giving rise to a noncompensatory pause following the JPC.

If conduction of the depolarization wave to the atria occurs more rapidly than conduction to the ventricles, then the inverted P wave will precede the QRS. If conduction to the atria occurs more slowly than conduction to the ventricles, then the inverted P wave will follow the QRS. If conduction of the depolarization wave occurs simultaneously to both the atria and ventricles then the inverted P wave will be hidden within the QRS complex.

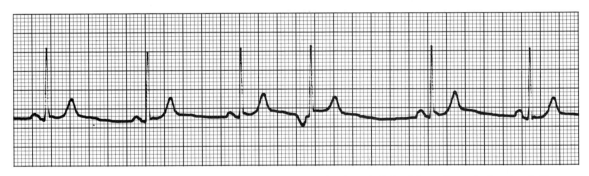

Sinus bradycardia with one isolated JPC with an inverted ectopic P wave.

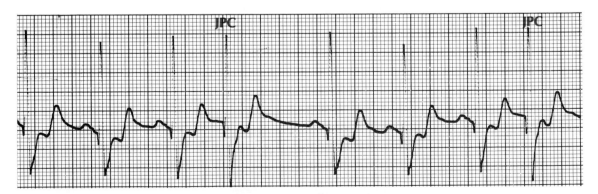

Sinus rhythm with bundle branch block and two isolated JPCs with no ectopic P waves demonstrated.

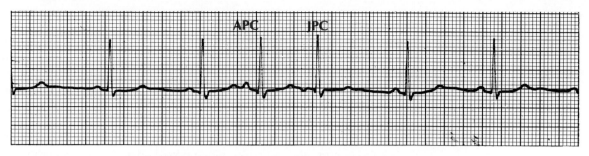

Sinus rhythm with one APC followed immediately by a JPC.

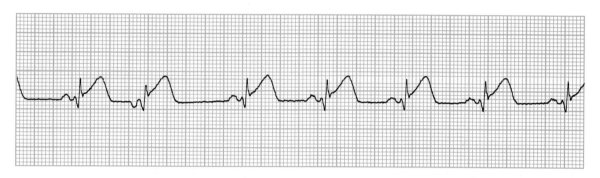

Sinus rhythm with ST elevation and one isolated JPC.

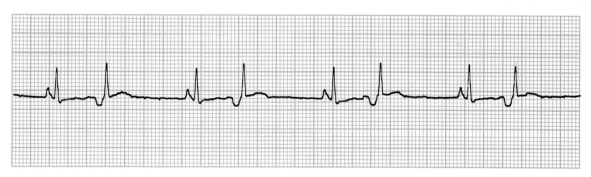

Sinus rhythm with JPCs in bigeminy.

VPCs

A VPC is a premature beat initiated in one area of the ventricles which depolarizes one ventricle and then with delay depolarizes the other ventricle through abnormal conduction pathways in the ventricular myocardium. This produces a wide and bizarre looking QRS complex .12 second or greater with a compensatory pause following it. Normally, the depolarization wave does not travel retrogradely to the atria, so the sinus P wave cycle is usually unaffected by the VPC. The sinus P wave continues on uninterrupted and occurs after the pause when expected and can sometimes be observed in the T wave of the VPC.

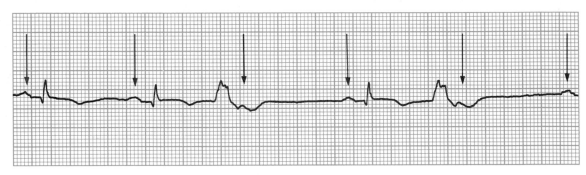

Sinus bradycardia with two isolated unifocal VPCs. The sinus P wave cycle continues on undisturbed by the VPCs. Arrows identify sinus P waves.

Types of Premature Contractions

A VPC may be **interpolated**—sandwiched between two sinus beats with no ventricular pause present. This is caused by the undisturbed sinus P wave falling outside the refractory period of the VPC and being able to be conducted to the ventricles and produce a normal QRS. Normally the sinus P wave is buried within the VPC or falls in its T wave. But when slow sinus rates occur the sinus P wave often falls after the T wave allowing normal conduction to occur.

INTERPOLATED VPC

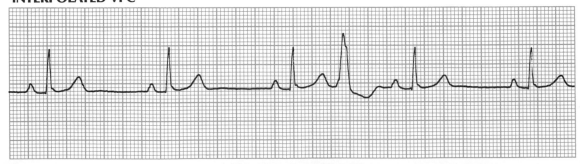

Sinus bradycardia with one interpolated VPC.

A VPC may be **malignant**—falling on the T wave of the previous beat and making the heart vulnerable to repetitive erratic heart beats.

A VPC may be **end diastolic**—occurring directly after a sinus P wave (end of diastole) before normal conduction to the ventricles occurs.

MALIGNANT VPC

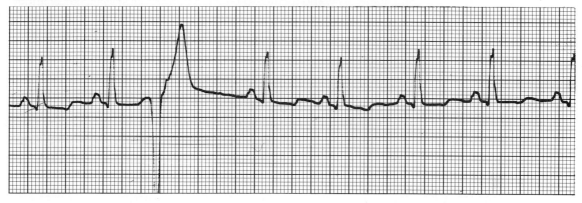

Sinus rhythm with one malignant VPC.

END DIASTOLIC VPC

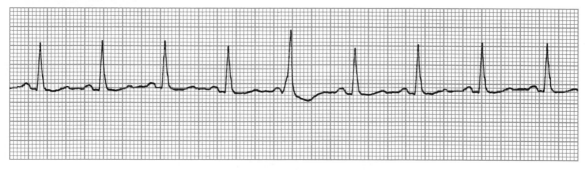

Sinus rhythm with one end diastolic VPC.

End diastolic VPCs arrive immediately after or occur while the sinus P waves are being inscribed and record a partially or completely formed sinus P wave followed immediately by a VPC. If the end diastolic VPC arrives after the sinus P wave has been fully formed, a **fusion beat** may occur. A fusion beat is a combination of both the end diastolic VPC and the sinus beat. The electrical activity in both the SA node and the ventricles occurs almost simultaneously, and the fusion beat is a combination of electrical impulses from both chambers and is a mixture in configuration of both the sinus QRS and the VPC and usually measures less than .12 second in duration.

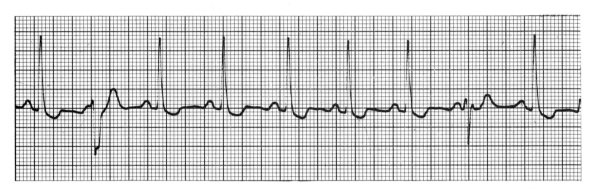

Sinus rhythm with two unifocal VPCs—the second is a fusion beat.

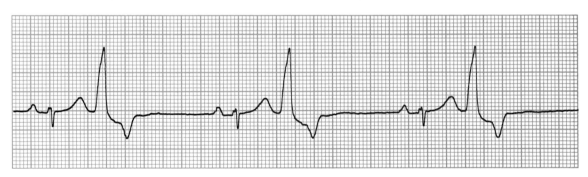

Sinus rhythm with unifocal VPCs in bigeminy.

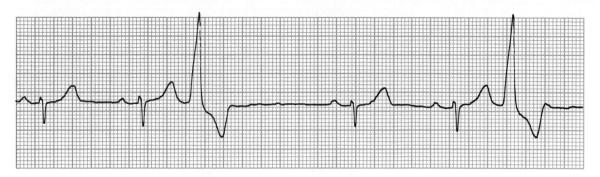

Sinus bradycardia with unifocal VPCs in trigeminy.

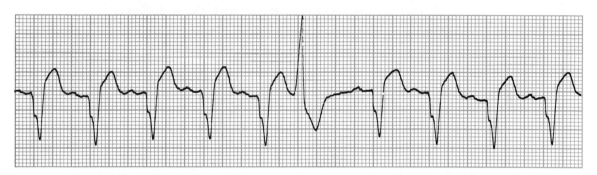

Sinus rhythm with bundle branch block and one isolated VPC.

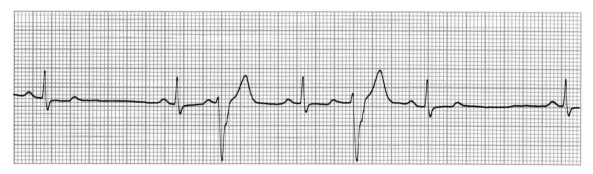

Sinus bradycardia with two unifocal interpolated VPCs.

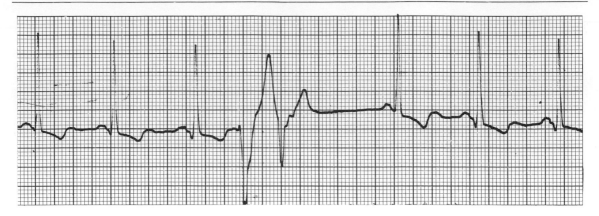

Sinus rhythm with a pair of VPCs—the second VPC is malignant.

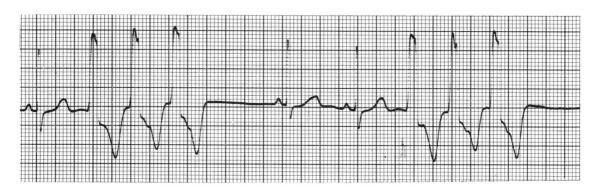

Sinus rhythm with two episodes of unifocal VPC triplets.

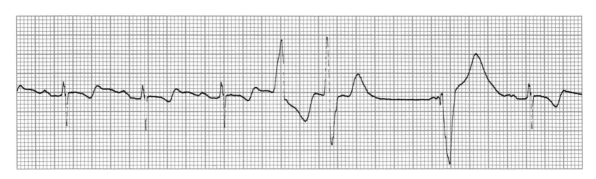

Sinus rhythm with first degree AV block and a pair of multifocal VPCs followed by a ventricular escape beat.

Differential Diagnosis

At this stage of the game VPCs are easy to distinguish from APCs and JPCs because of the wide and bizarre QRS complex that allows it to stand out from the rest of the rhythm. Resist the temptation to merely point out the VPC without following the interpretive steps previously outlined.

APCs and JPCs can often be difficult to distinguish from one another when their ectopic P waves become distorted or if they are superimposed on previous T waves. If interpretation is unclear, the term **supraventricular premature contraction** can be used to designate the more benign APC or JPC whose focus is located above the ventricles from the VPC.

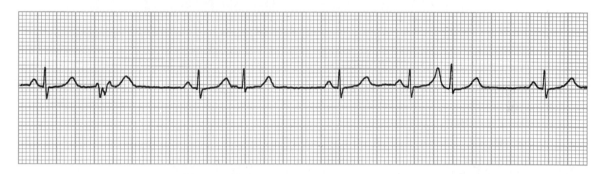

Sinus rhythm with one VPC and two isolated APCs. The VPC is easily distinguished from the APCs by its wide and bizarre QRS complex.

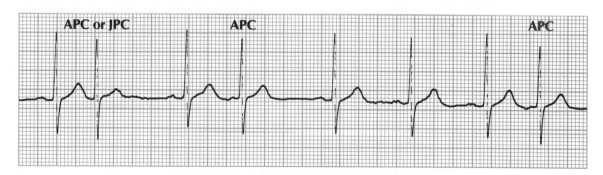

Sinus rhythm with three supraventricular premature contractions. The second and third premature beats are preceded by upright ectopic P waves indicating APCs. The first premature beat could have an upright ectopic P wave hidden in the T wave or could be a JPC with no ectopic P wave.

Nonconducted APCs and sinus arrhythmia can be a difficult differential diagnosis because both produce ventricular pauses. Sinus arrhythmia usually displays a gradual slowing and increase in the heart rate with the waxing and waning of respiration rather than the abrupt pause associated with nonconducted APCs. Although the most common cause of a pause is a nonconducted APC, you must be able to identify the ectopic P wave before you can make the diagnosis. Always check the previous T wave for hidden ectopic P waves.

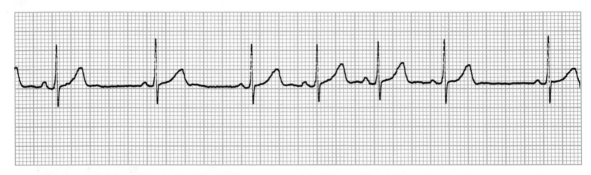

This strip demonstrates the increase and decrease in heart rate associated with sinus arrhythmia.

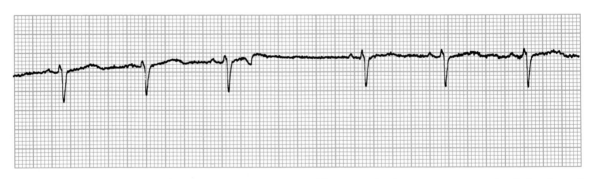

Sinus rhythm is present with a ventricular pause. No gradual slowing of the heart rate is present which is usually seen in sinus arrhythmia and there is a clear cut ectopic P wave buried in the T wave before the pause, confirming the diagnosis of a nonconducted APC.

Frequent APCs on a rhythm strip depict short R-R cycles, representing the APCs, and long R-R cycles representing the pauses following the APCs. These long and short cycles mimic the long and short R-R cycles found with sinus arrhythmia. But sinus arrhythmia will display constant PR intervals and no variation in the P wave configuration unlike APCs which display different looking ectopic P waves and varying PR intervals throughout the strip.

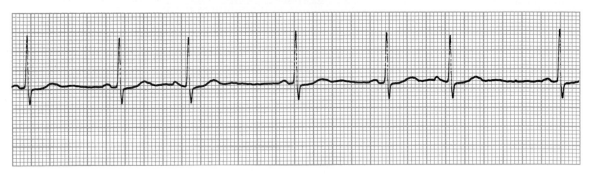

Although the heart rate slows and speeds up alternately suggesting sinus arrhythmia, the third and sixth P waves are early and configurations differ from the sinus P waves, confirming sinus rhythm with two isolated APCs.

PRACTICE ECGs

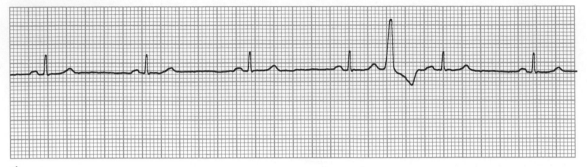

1

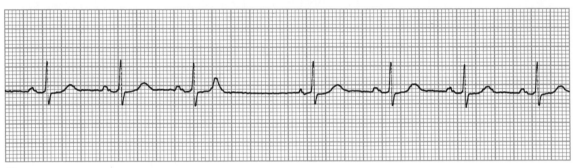

2

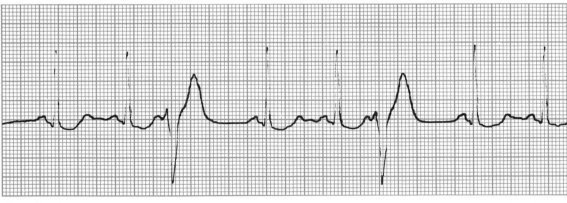

3

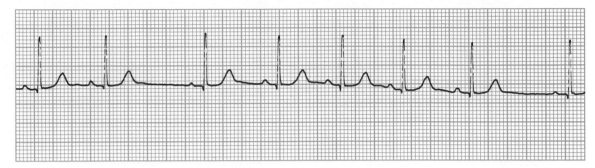

4

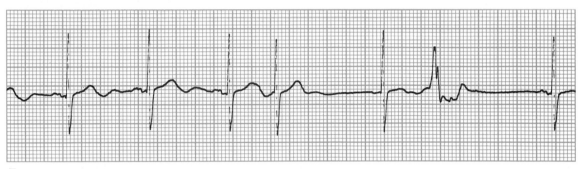

5

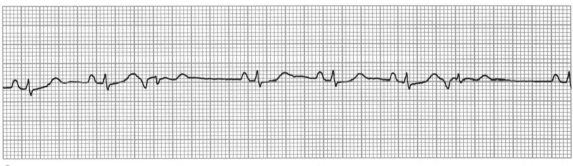

6

PRACTICE ECGs

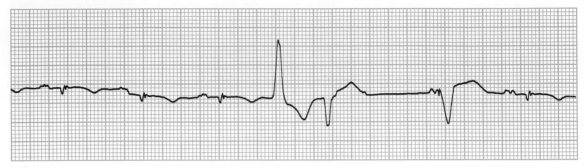

7

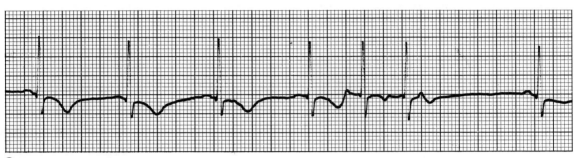

8

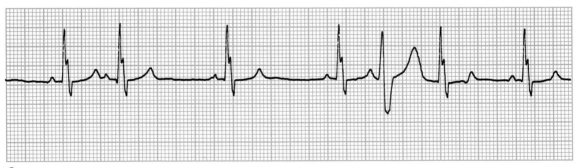

9

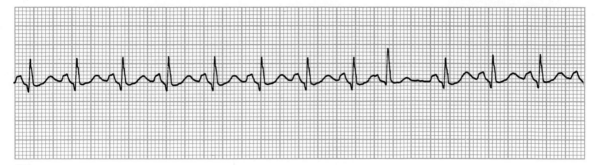

10

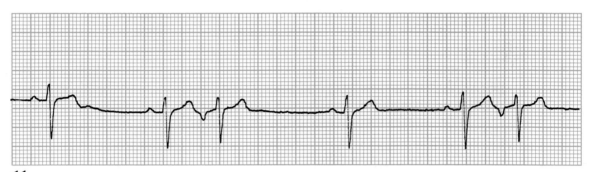

11

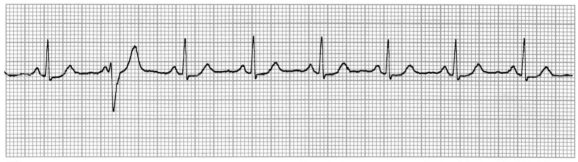

12

PRACTICE ECGs

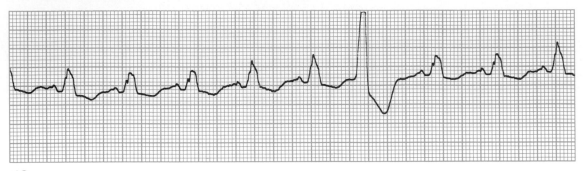

13

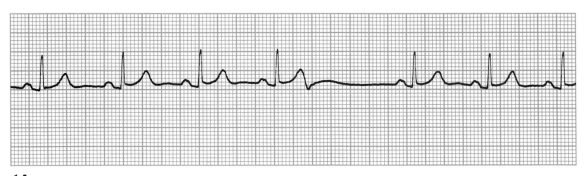

14

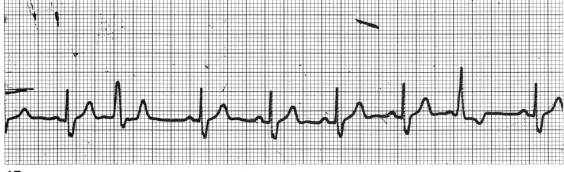

15

Answers To Practice ECGs

1. Sinus bradycardia with one interpolated VPC
2. Sinus rhythm with one nonconducted APC
3. Sinus rhythm with two unifocal VPCs in trigeminy
4. Sinus arrhythmia
5. Sinus rhythm with an isolated APC and VPC
6. Sinus rhythm with two isolated JPCs
7. Sinus rhythm with a pair of multifocal VPCs followed by a ventricular escape beat
8. Sinus rhythm with three APCs in a row with the last APC nonconducted
9. Sinus arrhythmia with bundle branch block and an isolated APC and an interpolated VPC
10. Sinus tachycardia with one isolated APC
11. Sinus bradycardia with two isolated JPCs
12. Sinus rhythm with one end diastolic VPC
13. Sinus rhythm with bundle branch block and one isolated VPC
14. Sinus rhythm with one nonconducted APC
15. Sinus rhythm with two multifocal VPCs—the second is end diastolic

ATRIAL RHYTHMS

Atrial Tachycardia (Paroxysmal Atrial Tachycardia)

Multifocal Atrial Tachycardia

Atrial Flutter

Atrial Fibrillation

Differential Diagnosis

Practice ECGs

Practice ECG Answers

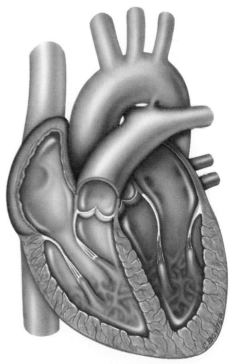

Paroxysmal Atrial Tachycardia

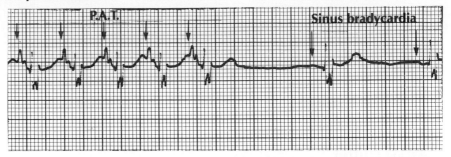

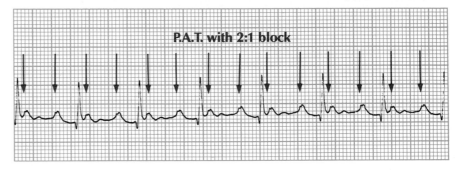

CRITERIA

1. 4-6 or more unifocal APCs in a row with a regular P-P cycle between 140-220/min.

2. QRS resembles that of the regular cardiac rhythm

3. If the atrial rhythm is rapid all of the ectopic P waves may not be conducted to the ventricles (PAT with block)

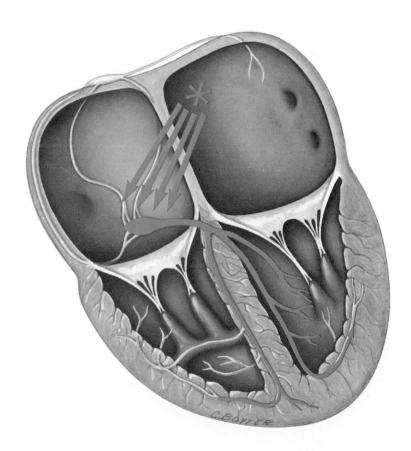

ATRIAL RHYTHMS

Multifocal Atrial Tachycardia

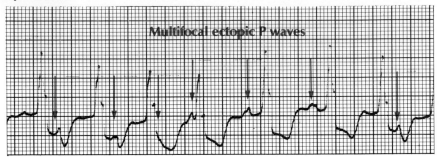

CRITERIA

1. **4-6 multifocal APCS in a row with an irregular P-P cycle, varying PR intervals, at a rate between 100-200/min.**

2. **Varying P wave configurations**

3. **Some APCs may be nonconducted**

4. **QRS resembles that of the regular cardiac rhythm**

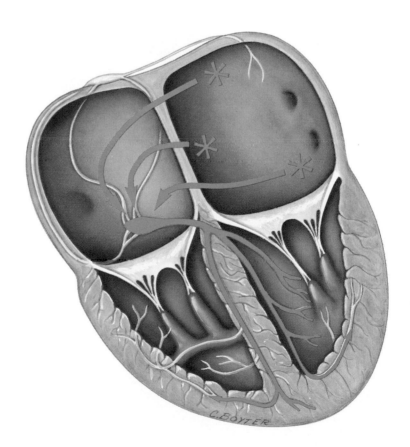

ATRIAL RHYTHMS

Atrial Flutter

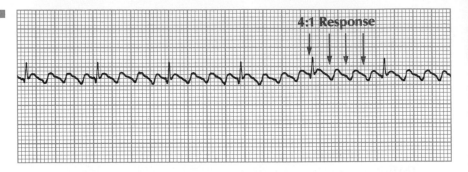

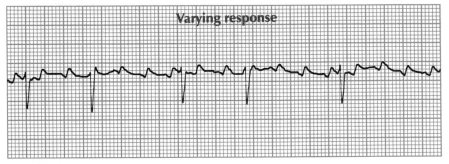

CRITERIA

1. **One ectopic focus in the atria fires repeatedly at a rate between 220-350/min.**

2. **Flutter waves replace P waves**

3. **QRS resembles that of the regular cardiac rhythm**

4. **Ventricular response can be 1:1, 2:1, 3:1, etc., or can vary**

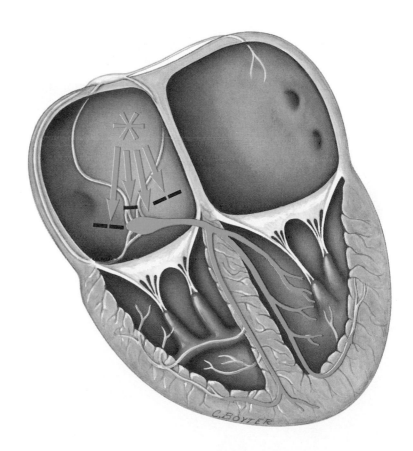

ATRIAL RHYTHMS

Atrial Fibrillation

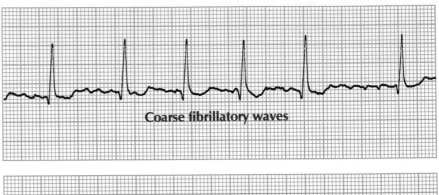

Coarse fibrillatory waves

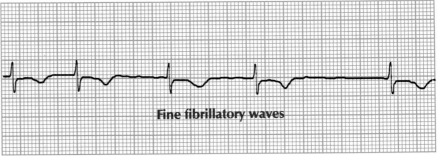

Fine fibrillatory waves

CRITERIA

1. **Multifocal ectopic foci in the atria fire repeatedly at a rate between 350-650/min.**

2. **Fibrillatory waves, either coarse or fine, replace P waves**

3. **Ventricular response is extremely irregular**

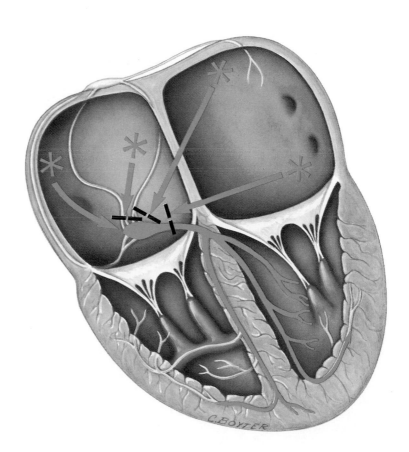

Atrial rhythms originate in an area of the atria anywhere other than the SA node and are composed of at least 4-6 ectopic beats in a row. They are categorized by atrial configuration and atrial rate. Conduction to the ventricles follows normal conduction pathways recording QRS complexes that resemble those of the dominant rhythm. During these atrial rhythms, it is the foci in the atria that are depolarizing at the rapid rate and the ventricles may or may not respond to each ectopic atrial depolarization. If the ventricles respond to every ectopic atrial depolarization it is called 1:1 conduction—one P wave for each QRS.

During rapid atrial rates over 180 beats per minute, the ventricles often respond to only every other or every few atrial depolarizations. As the atrial depolarization wave travels to the AV node it finds that it is refractory from the previous beat and unable to transmit the next depolarization wave when it arrives. This refractoriness displayed by the conduction system prevents the ventricles from depolarizing and contracting too rapidly and producing a rapid heart rate with an inadequate systemic blood flow. This safety mechanism functions in most instances—but not all the time.

If the atrial rate is very rapid and it is impossible to distinguish which atrial rhythm is operating, the term **superventricular tachycardia** is acceptable.

Atrial Tachycardia (Paroxysmal Atrial Tachycardia)

Paroxysmal atrial tachycardia (PAT) is a run of 4-6 or more APCs in a row with a regular or slightly irregular P-P cycle at a rate between 140-220 beats per minute and 1:1 conduction with the ventricles. In short bursts of atrial tachycardia the P-P cycle may be more irregular. If the atrial rate is too rapid the ventricles may not be able to respond to every ectopic P wave and PAT with block will occur. This prevents the ventricles from depolarizing and contracting too rapidly.

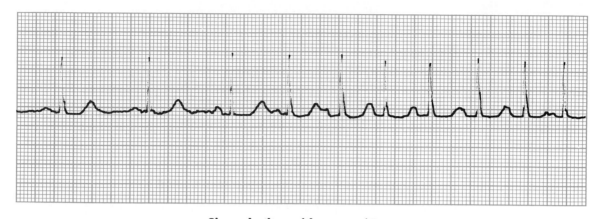

Sinus rhythm with a run of PAT.

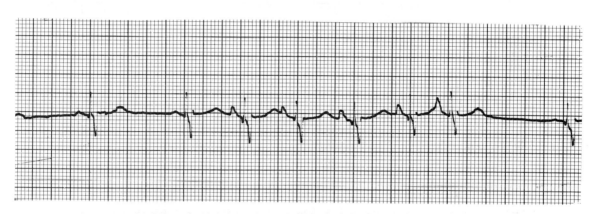

Sinus bradycardia with a short burst of PAT with a return
to sinus bradycardia.

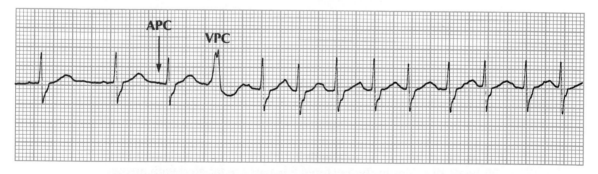

Sinus rhythm with an isolated APC and VPC and a run of PAT.

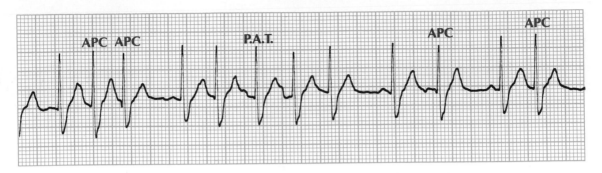

Sinus rhythm with two isolated APCs, a pair of APCs and a short burst of PAT.

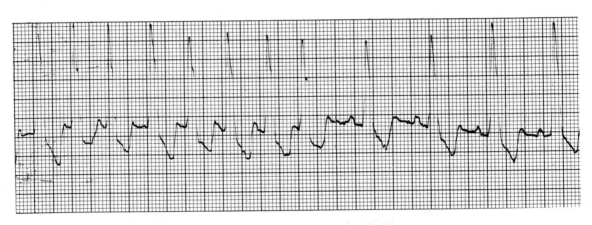

PAT followed by sinus rhythm with bundle branch block.

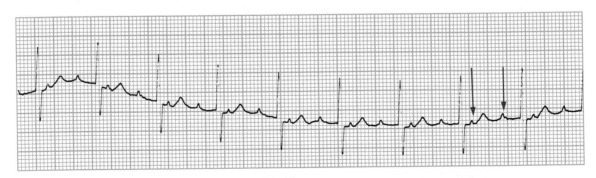

PAT at 190 beats per minute with 2:1 block and a ventricular rate of 95 beats per minute. Two ectopic P waves are labeled with arrows.

DIFFERENTIAL DIAGNOSIS OF ARRHYTHMIAS

Multifocal Atrial Tachycardia (MAT)

MAT is a run of 4-6 or more multifocal APCs in a row with irregular P-P cycles and varying PR intervals at a rate between 100-200 beats per minute with 1:1 conduction with the ventricles. Because the APCs are multifocal in origin, the PR intervals vary from focus to focus and the P wave configurations show variation. The ectopic P waves are often peaked and tent-shaped. Some of the APCs may be nonconducted to the ventricles.

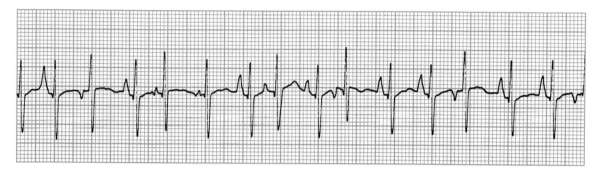

Multifocal atrial tachycardia.

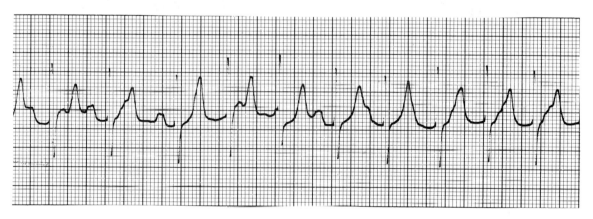

Multifocal atrial tachycardia.

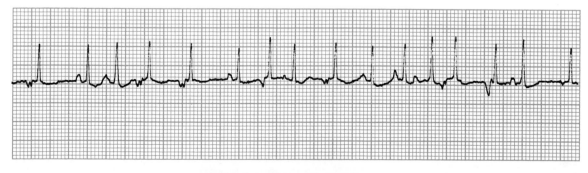

Multifocal atrial tachycardia.

Atrial Flutter

One theory of impulse formation in atrial flutter is that one ectopic focus in the atria depolarizes at a regular rate between 220-350 beats per minute. The flutter waves are usually regular in untreated atrial flutter and may be slightly irregular following drug therapy or very irregular during short bursts of atrial flutter. Because of the rapid atrial rate **flutter waves** replace P waves on an ECG and display a sawtooth configuration. The prominent negative component of the sawtooth configuration is said to represent the Ta wave on the ECG and appears opposite to that of the P wave. The flutter waves distort QRS complexes, ST segments, and T waves as they occur at a rapid, regular rate.

The physiological refractoriness of the AV node prevents the ventricles from responding to all the flutter waves and produces 2:1, 3:1, 4:1, etc. or a varying ventricular response. This lack of 1:1 conduction protects the ventricles from depolarizing too rapidly and compromising the systemic circulation. One of the concerns with the establishment of atrial flutter in a patient is that 1:1 conduction may occur and cause an emergency situation as the ventricles respond at 300 per minute.

Flutter waves are difficult to distinguish when the ventricular response is 2:1. There are only two flutter waves for each QRS complex and they are often superimposed on the ST segments and T waves making identification difficult. Try turning the tracing upside down to visualize the flutter waves. A 3:1 or greater conduction ratio slows the ventricular rate to allow the flutter waves to become clearly visible in between QRS complexes.

After atrial flutter has been diagnosed calculate both the atrial and ventricular rate. Atrial flutter at 300 per minute indicates that the atria are depolarizing at 300 per minute—not the ventricles. Calculate the ventricular rate and establish a conduction ratio (2:1, 3:1, etc.) in order to complete the interpretation.

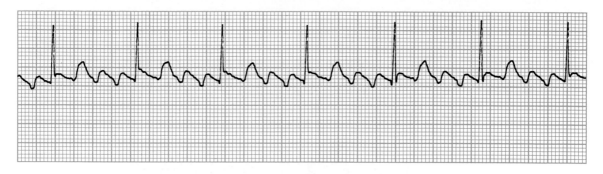

**Atrial flutter at 280 beats per minute with 4:1 conduction and a
ventricular rate of 70 beats per minute.**

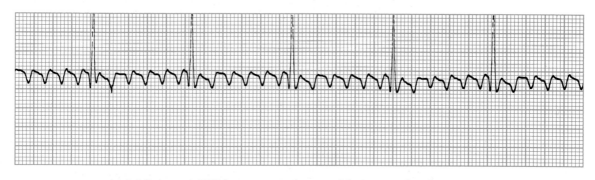

**Atrial flutter at 336 beats per minute with 6:1 conduction and a
ventricular rate of 56 beats per minute.**

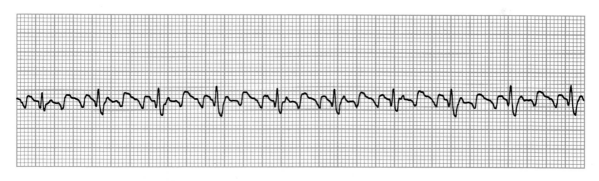

**Atrial flutter at 300 beats per minute with 3:1 conduction and a
ventricular rate of 100 beats per minute.**

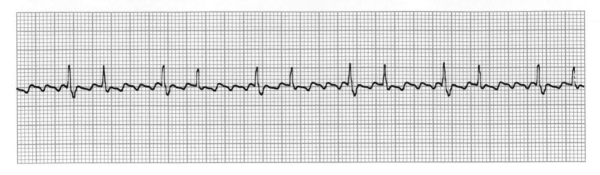

Atrial flutter at 375 beats per minute with a variable conduction and an average ventricular response of 125 beats per minute.

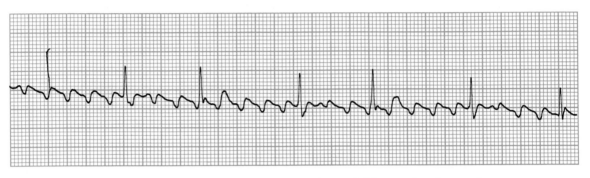

Atrial flutter at 300 beats per minute with variable conduction and an average ventricular response of 67 beats per minute.

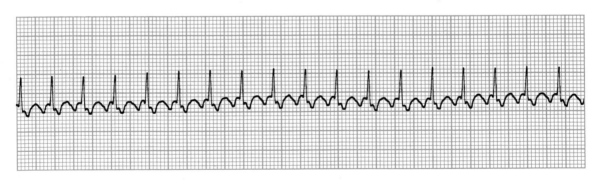

Atrial flutter at 350 beats per minute with 2:1 conduction and a ventricular rate of 175 beats per minute.

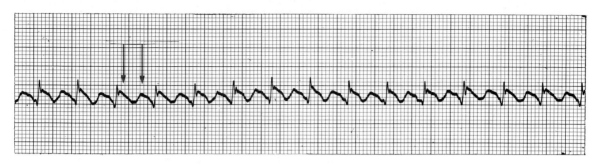

Atrial flutter at 300 beats per minute with 2:1 conduction and a ventricular response of 150 beats per minute. Two flutter waves are labeled with arrows.

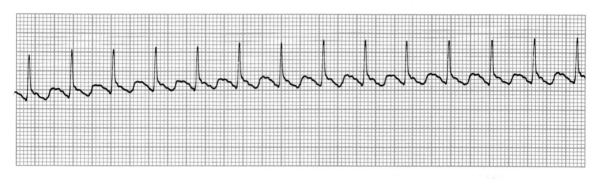

Atrial flutter at 270 beats per minute with 2:1 conduction and a ventricular rate of 135 beats per minute.

Atrial Fibrillation

One theory of impulse formation in atrial fibrillation is that multifocal ectopic foci in the atria fire repeatedly at a rate between 350-650 per minute. Because of the extremely rapid atrial rate **fibrillatory waves,** either coarse or fine, replace P waves. One ectopic focus fires immediately after another giving rise to a quivering in the atria rather than contractions.

The AV node is constantly rendered refractory by the hundreds of fibrillatory waves each minute allowing only sporadic depolarization impulses to be conducted to the ventricles to produce QRS complexes. The ventricular response recorded is irregularly, irregular.

A rapid ventricular response often mimics ventricular regularity and leads to an erroneous interpretation. Slow ventricular rates accentuate ventricular irregularity— rapid ventricular rates mask ventricular irregularity. Make careful observations and measurements.

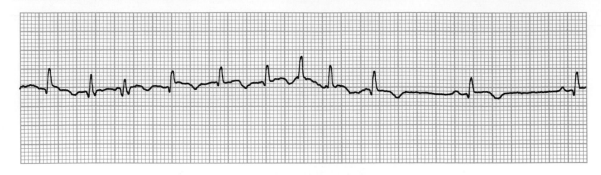

Atrial fibrillation with a rapid ventricular response converting to sinus bradycardia.

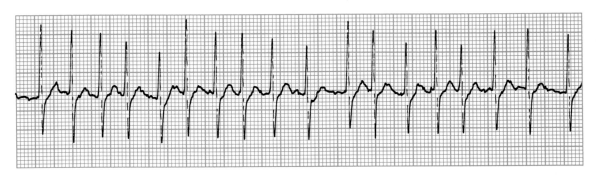

Atrial fibrillation with a rapid ventricular response initially mimicking ventricular regularity as in PAT. But careful observation reveals variable R-R cycles confirming atrial fibrillation.

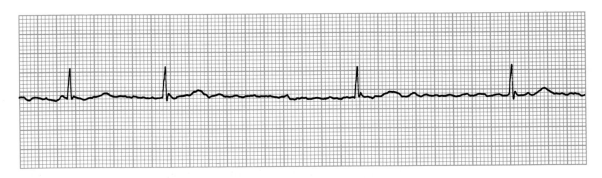

Atrial fibrillation with a slow ventricular response.

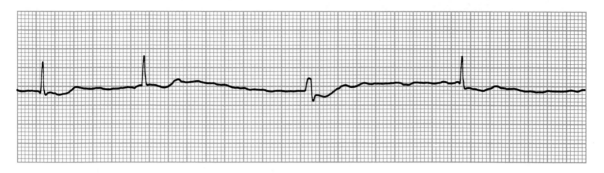

Atrial fibrillation with a slow ventricular response and a ventricular escape beat terminating a long ventricular pause.

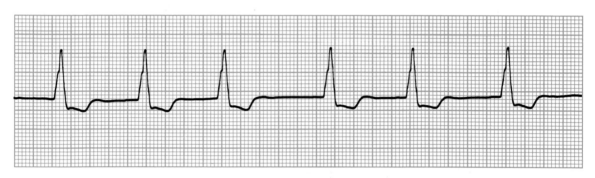

Atrial fibrillation with bundle branch block.

Differential Diagnosis

In distinguishing between different atrial rhythms, make an initial overall assessment of the strip. Are P waves present? Are PR intervals regular? Are flutter waves or fibrillatory waves in evidence? Is the ventricular rate regular or does it vary? Then make some assumptions. Ventricular rates can be regular with PAT and atrial flutter—but P waves will occur with PAT and flutter waves with atrial flutter. Although the P waves associated with PAT with block may sometimes resemble the configuration of flutter waves, calculate the atrial rate and be sure that it fits the criteria for diagnosis. The atrial rate for PAT is 140-220 beats per minute and 220-350 beats per minute for atrial flutter.

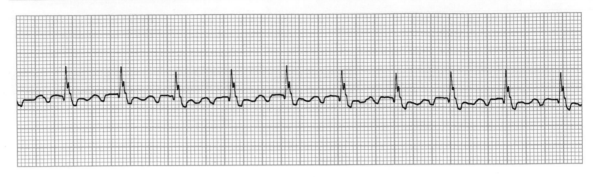

Although this appears to be atrial flutter with 2:1 conduction, the atrial rate is 210 beats per minute establishing the diagnosis of PAT with 2:1 conduction.

Ventricular rates will be irregular with MAT and atrial fibrillation—but multifocal P waves will be recorded with MAT and fibrillatory waves with atrial fibrillation.

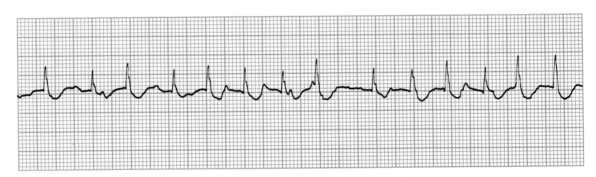

On initial observation, atrial fibrillation is suggested by the very irregular ventricular response and lack of sinus P waves. But multifocal ectopic P waves can be identified confirming the diagnosis of multifocal atrial tachycardia.

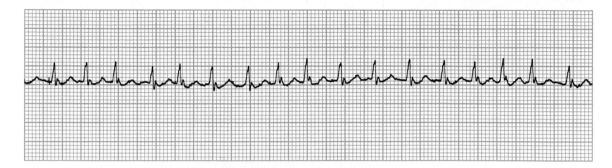

Atrial fibrillation with a rapid ventricular response. What appear to be multifocal ectopic P waves preceding each QRS are T waves, ruling out the diagnosis of multifocal atrial tachycardia.

PAT with block and MAT both have P waves and irregular ventricular rates—but PAT demonstrates unifocal P waves and constant PR intervals and MAT exhibits multifocal P waves and varying PR intervals.

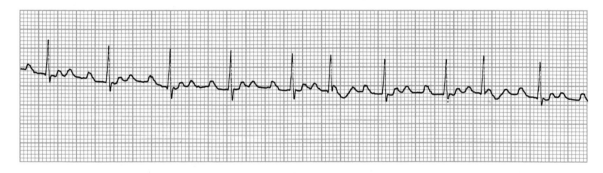

PAT with varying conduction. The ectopic P waves are all identical in configuration, ruling out the diagnosis of multifocal atrial tachycardia.

Atrial fibrillation with a rapid ventricular response can easily be mistaken for atrial tachycardia. The R-R cycle appears to regularize with rapid ventricular rates. Always measure—never assume rates are regular.

It is impossible to distinguish sinus tachycardia from atrial tachycardia from a single six second rhythm strip. Both rhythms demonstrate P waves and rates above 100 beats per minute. There's no way to distinguish a sinus P wave from an ectopic atrial P wave without having a rhythm strip demonstrating exactly how the increase in rate occurred. Was it a gradual increase in rate accompanied by an activity signifying a sinus tachycardia or was it an abrupt increase in rate precipitated by an APC denoting atrial tachycardia?

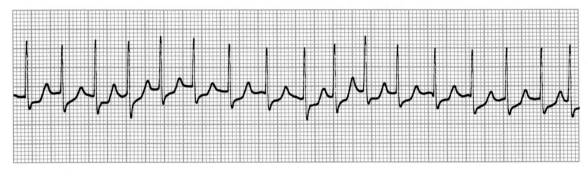

Atrial fibrillation with a rapid ventricular response of 170 beats per minute mimicking atrial tachycardia. The clue for correct diagnosis is the slight variation in the R-R cycles.

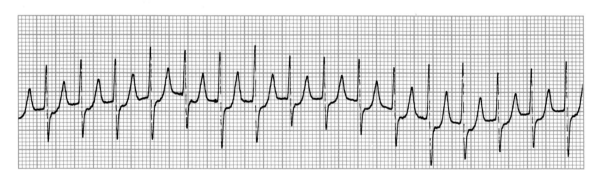

This is an example of atrial tachycardia, although without clinical correlation it is impossible to make a definite diagnosis from this short strip alone.

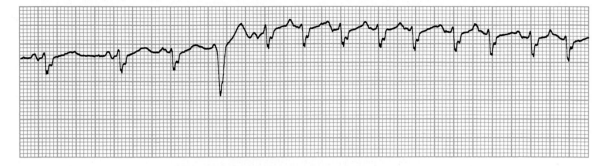

This strip allows one to make a definite diagnosis of PAT as the first beat of the tachycardia is visible and can be compared with the first two sinus beats in the strip. An isolated VPC is present after the first beat of the PAT.

During PAT with 2:1 block, every other ectopic P wave may be hidden in the T wave of a QRS and sinus rhythm may be diagnosed erroneously. Carefully evaluate the ST-T segments for any abnormal configurations and/or hidden waves.

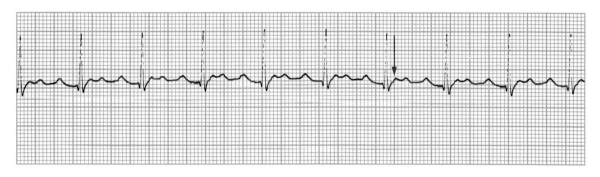

PAT at 187 beats per minute mimicking sinus rhythm. The second P wave is buried in the ST segment and labeled with an arrow.

Sometimes during sinus tachycardia the T waves may imitate a second ectopic atrial wave and lead to the diagnosis of atrial flutter. The measurement of T wave to P wave throughout an ECG strip normally will not present a regular measurement cycle and the T waves will display a different configuration than the P waves.

By making observations, taking measurements and comparing them to the criteria, interpretation becomes organized and less difficult. Arrhythmia interpretation is a game of simply ruling out possibilities until you're left with one or more viable interpretations.

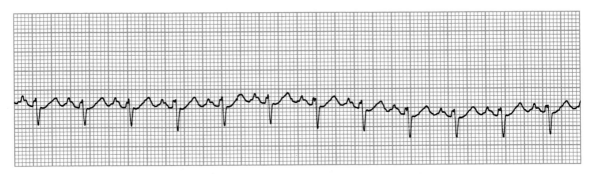

Sinus tachycardia imitating atrial flutter. On close examination all the sinus P waves are identical and do not resemble the T waves and the T to P cycle is not regular.

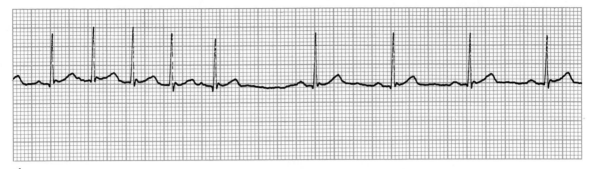

1

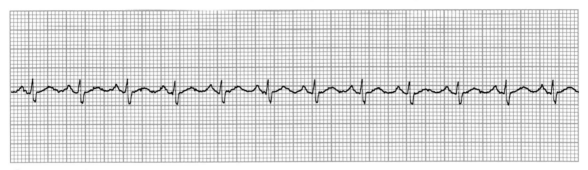

2

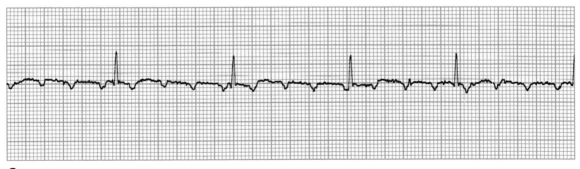

3

PRACTICE ECGs

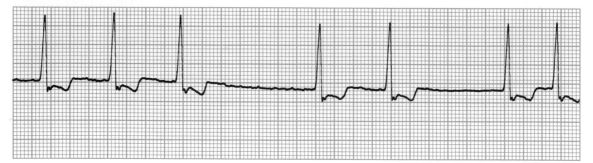

4

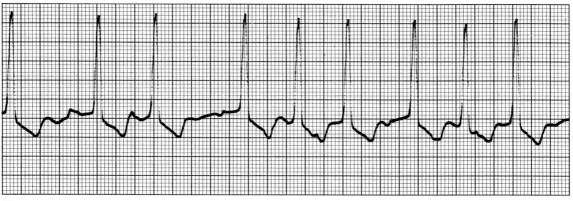

5

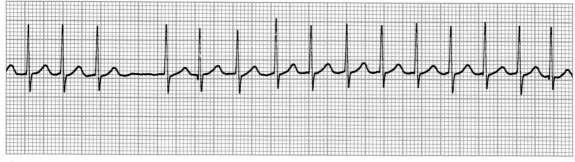

6

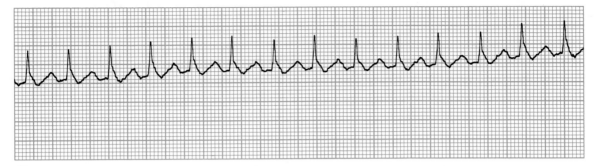

7

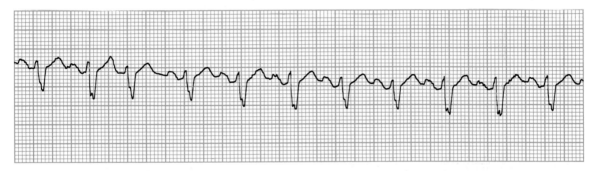

8

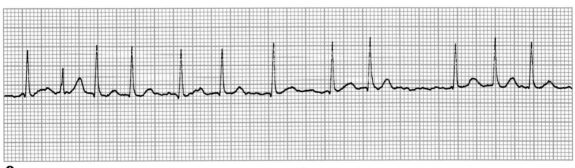

9

PRACTICE ECGs

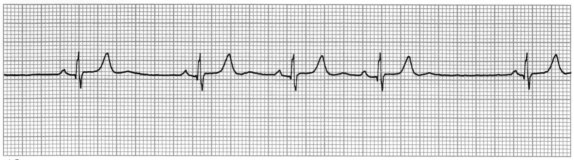

10

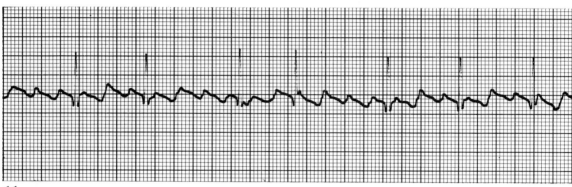

11

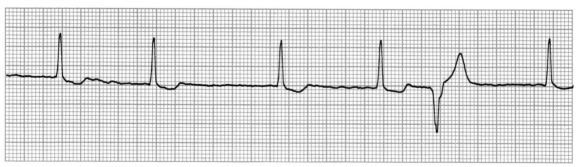

12

DIFFERENTIAL DIAGNOSIS OF ARRHYTHMIAS

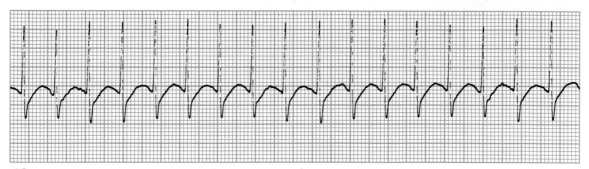

13

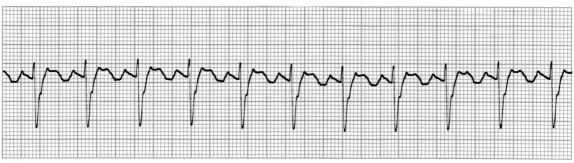

14

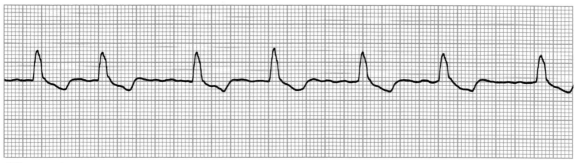

15

Practice ECG Answers

1. Short burst of PAT reverting to sinus rhythm
2. Sinus tachycardia
3. PAT with 4:1 conduction
4. Atrial fibrillation
5. Multifocal atrial tachycardia
6. Atrial fibrillation
7. Atrial flutter with 2:1 conduction
8. Sinus tachycardia with bundle branch block and one isolated APC
9. Atrial fibrillation
10. Sinus arrhythmia
11. Atrial flutter with variable conduction
12. Atrial fibrillation with one isolated VPC
13. Supraventricular tachycardia
14. Atrial flutter with 2:1 conduction and bundle branch block
15. Atrial fibrillation with bundle branch block

JUNCTIONAL RHYTHMS

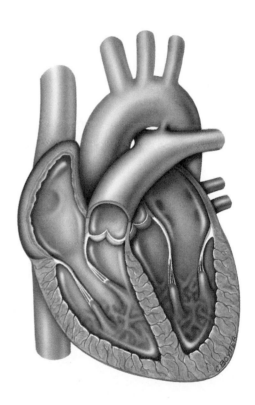

JUNCTIONAL RHYTHMS

Junctional Escape Rhythm

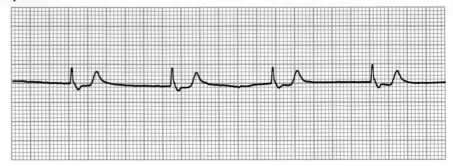

CRITERIA

1. 4-6 or more junctional escape beats in a row at a regular rate below 60/min.

2. QRS resembles that of the normal cardiac rhythm

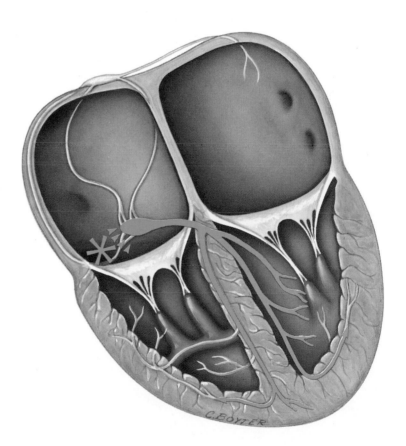

JUNCTIONAL RHYTHMS

Accelerated Junctional Rhythm

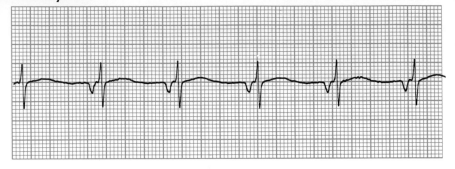

CRITERIA

1. 4-6 or more JPCs in a row at a regular rate between 60-100/min.

2. QRS resembles that of the normal cardiac rhythm

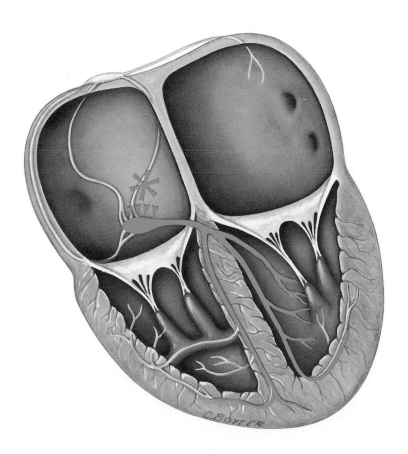

JUNCTIONAL RHYTHMS

JUNCTIONAL RHYTHMS

Junctional Tachycardia

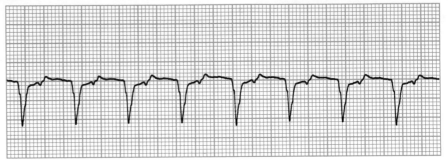

CRITERIA

1. **4-6 or more JPCs in a row 100/min.**

2. **QRS resembles that of the normal cardiac rhythm**

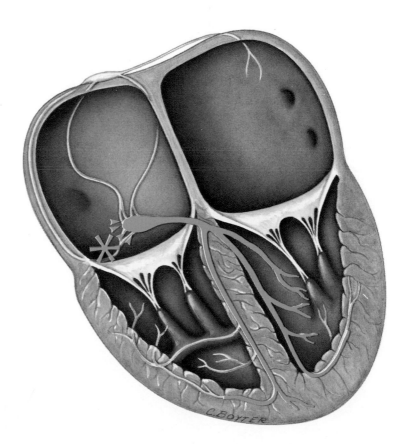

Junctional rhythms originate in an area around the AV junction and are composed of at least 4-6 ectopic beats in a row. Conduction to the ventricles follows normal conduction pathways recording QRS complexes that resemble those of the dominant cardiac rhythm.

Junctional rhythms are categorized by rate. Interpretation is fairly straightforward with the slow, regular ventricular rates accompanying junctional escape rhythms and accelerated junctional rhythms. Identifying ectopic inverted P waves preceding or following the QRS complexes or the absence of them is easy. It's only when the more rapid junctional tachycardias occur that identifying ectopic P waves becomes difficult.

During junctional rhythms a phenomenon called **AV dissociation** may occur where the atria are under the control of a separate pacemaking focus, usually the SA node, and the ventricles are controlled by one of the junctional rhythms. The two pacemaking foci, usually firing at fairly similar rates, temporarily coexist without disturbing one another because their impulses spread to the respective heart chambers almost simultaneously. If the atria are in sinus rhythm, the P waves float in to and out of the QRS complexes without bearing any relation to them.

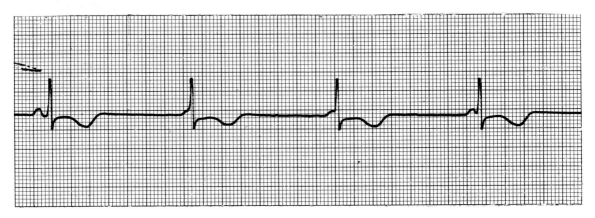

Sinus bradycardia with AV dissociation and a junctional escape rhythm.

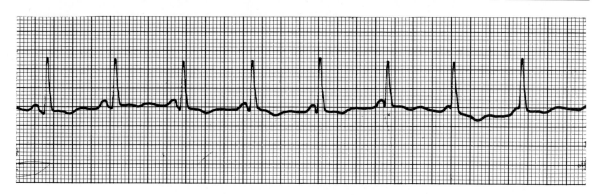

Sinus rhythm with AV dissociation and an accelerated junctional rhythm.

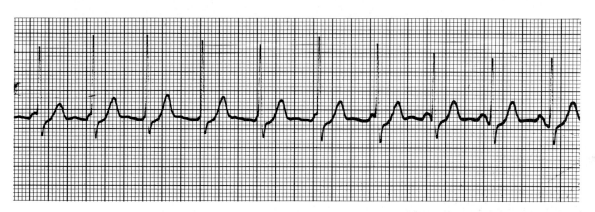

Sinus tachycardia with AV dissociation and junctional tachycardia.

Junctional Escape Rhythm

Is a run of 4-6 or more junctional escape beats in a row at a regular rate below 60 beats per minute. As with junctional escape beats, the inverted ectopic P wave can either precede, follow, or be lost within the QRS complex. Junctional escape rhythms save the heart from excessively slow heart rhythms or asystole. If the AV junction does not respond to long ventricular pauses, ventricular escape rhythms are the last line of defense. (Refer to Chapter 6)

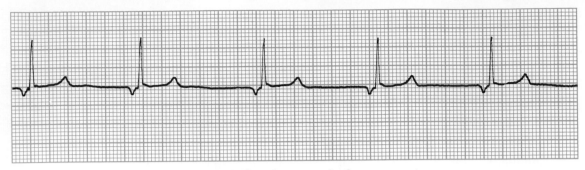

Junctional escape rhythm.

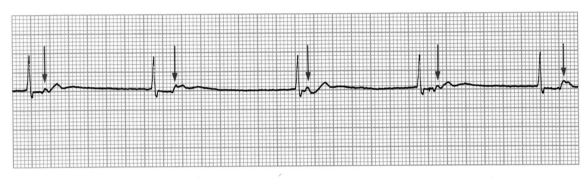

Sinus bradycardia with AV dissociation and a junctional escape rhythm.
Sinus P waves are labeled with arrows.

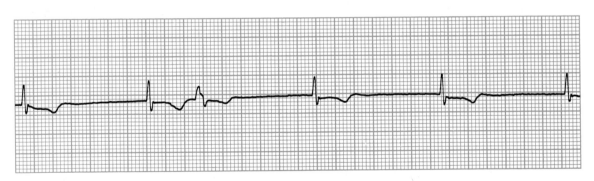

Junctional escape rhythm with one VPC.

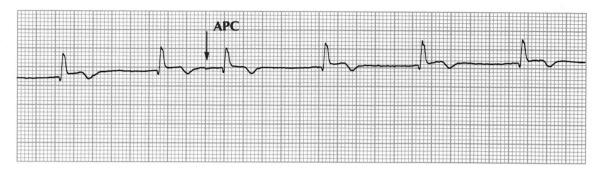

Junctional escape rhythm with one isolated APC.

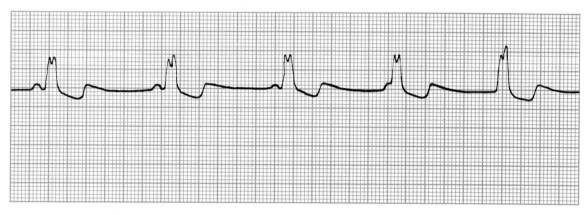

Sinus bradycardia with bundle branch block and AV dissociation and a junctional escape rhythm.

Accelerated Junctional Rhythm

Is a run of 4-6 or more junctional beats in a row at a regular rate between 60-100 beats per minute. Inverted ectopic P waves either precede, follow, or are buried within the QRS complexes.

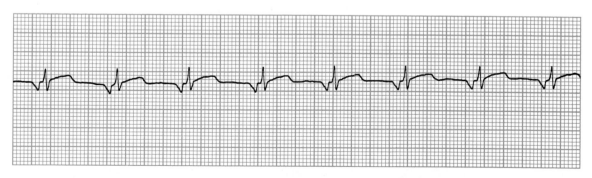

Accelerated junctional rhythm.

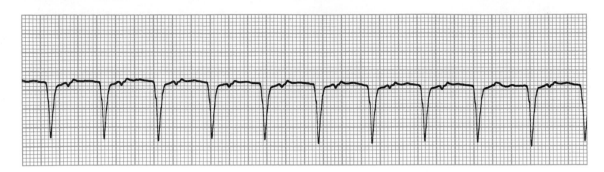

**Accelerated junctional rhythm. Inverted ectopic P waves are buried
in the T waves.**

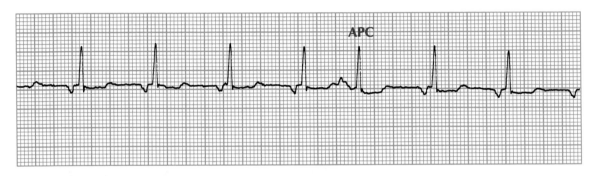

Accelerated junctional rhythm with one isolated APC.

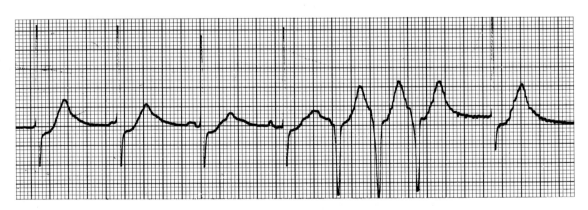

**Sinus rhythm with AV dissociation and an accelerated junctional rhythm
with three unifocal VPCs in a row.**

Junctional Tachycardia

Is a run of 4-6 or more JPCs in a row at a regular rate over 100 beats per minute. Inverted ectopic P waves either precede, follow, or are buried within the QRS complexes.

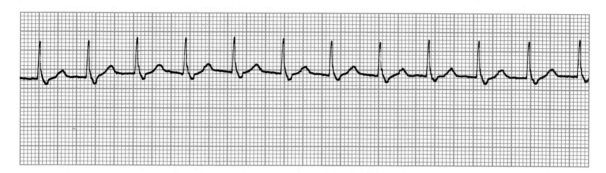

Junctional tachycardia.

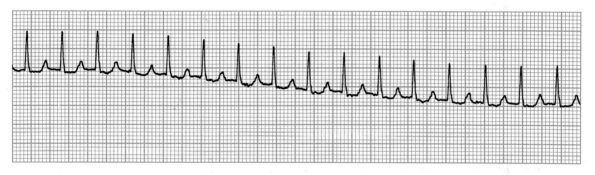

Junctional tachycardia.

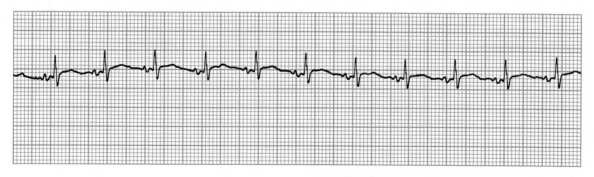

Junctional tachycardia.

Differential Diagnosis

Rapid ventricular rates can make differentiating between atrial rhythms and junctional rhythms a challenge at best—an impossibility at worst. The inverted ectopic P waves of a junctional tachycardia or the lack of them, and the upright ectopic P waves of an atrial tachycardia become superimposed on the T waves and make proper identification impossible when ventricular rates are rapid. When this occurs, the term supraventricular tachycardia is used and denotes an inability to specifically identify a rhythm above the ventricles.

Atrial flutter with 2:1 conduction can initially be mistaken for a junctional tachycardia. The saw tooth configuration of the second flutter wave closest to the QRS mimics the inverted P wave of a junctional tachycardia. The first flutter wave is superimposed on the ST segment or T wave of the previous QRS. If the conduction ratio of the atrial flutter is 3:1 or 4:1 identifying the flutter waves is easy. In a rhythm strip that first appears to be a junctional rhythm, always examine the ST segments and T waves for hidden flutter waves.

Atrial fibrillation with fine fibrillatory waves and a slow ventricular response may simulate a junctional escape rhythm with no visible ectopic P waves. The ventricular irregularity accompanying a slow ventricular response with atrial fibrillation should allow you to rule out a junctional escape rhythm which should display a fairly regular R-R cycle.

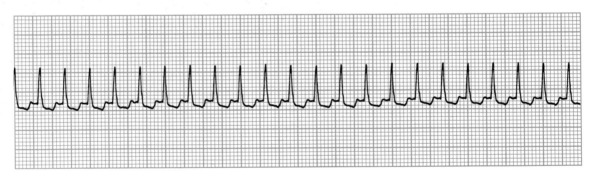

Supraventricular tachycardia.

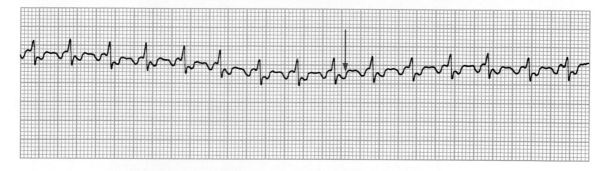

Atrial flutter at 300 beats per minute with 2:1 conduction and a
ventricular rate of 150 beats per minute. At first glance this strip
resembles a junctional tachycardia with an inverted P wave preceding
each QRS. But a second ectopic wave (identified with an arrow) is buried
in each ST segment confirming atrial flutter.

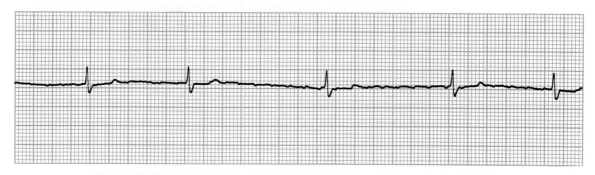

Atrial fibrillation with a slow ventricular response simulating a junctional
escape rhythm. The R-R cycle displays variation and therefore rules out
a junctional escape rhythm.

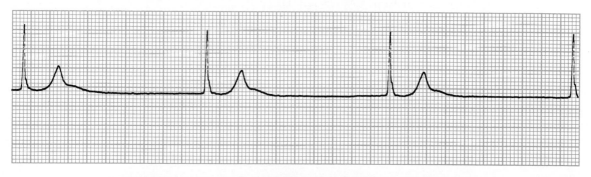

Junctional escape rhythm with a regular R-R cycle ruling out
atrial fibrillation.

During sinus rhythm with marked first degree AV block, the sinus P waves may move far enough leftward to become superimposed on the previous T wave and an erroneous interpretation of junctional rhythm may be made. Always scrutinize the T waves for any abnormal configurations or waves.

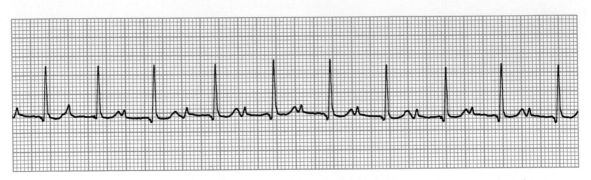

Sinus rhythm with marked first degree AV block mimicking an accelerated junctional rhythm. The sinus P wave is located on the downslope of the T wave.

PRACTICE ECGs

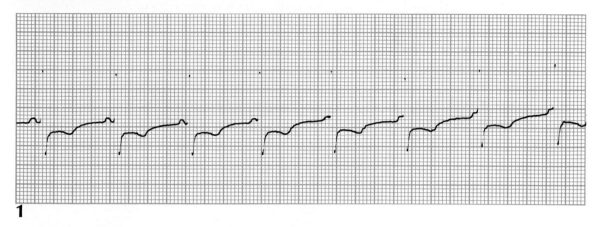

1

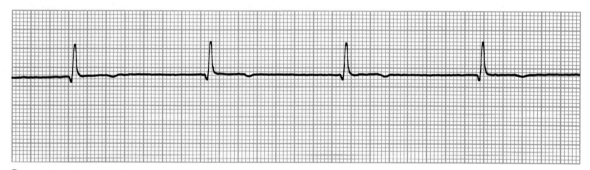

2

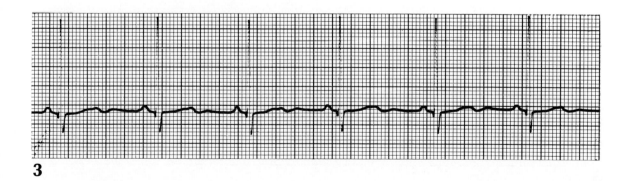

3

JUNCTIONAL RHYTHMS

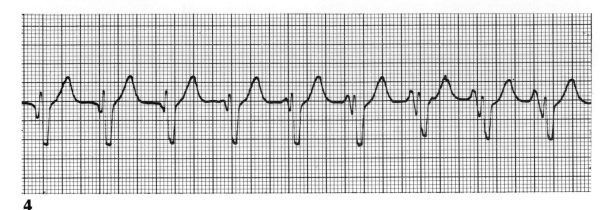

4

5

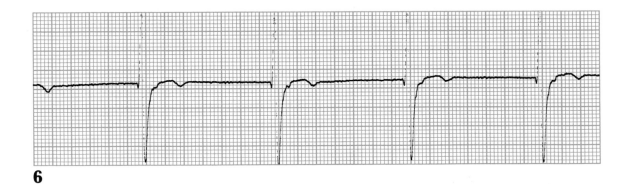

6

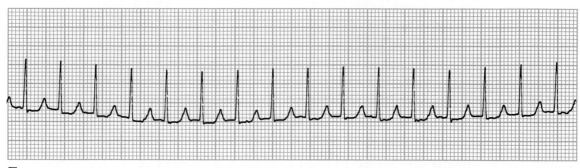

7

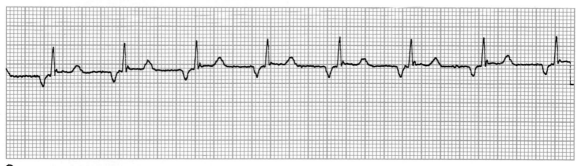

8

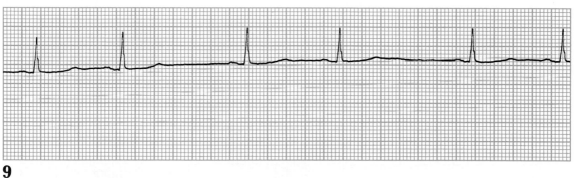

9

PRACTICE ECGs

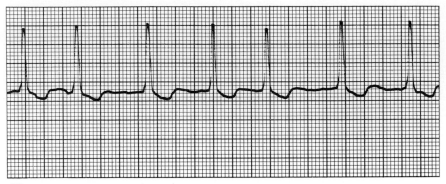

10

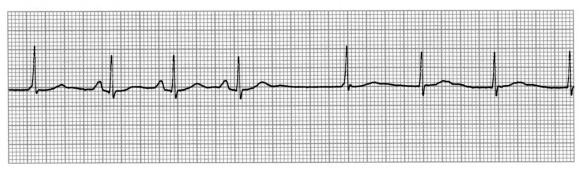

11

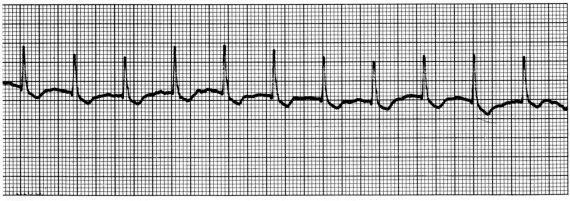

12

DIFFERENTIAL DIAGNOSIS OF ARRHYTHMIAS

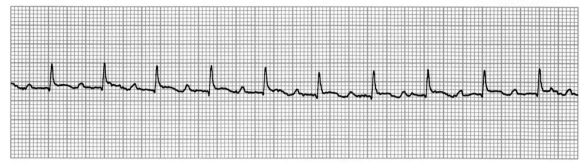

13

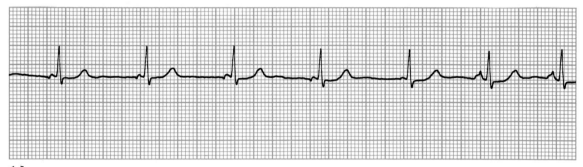

14

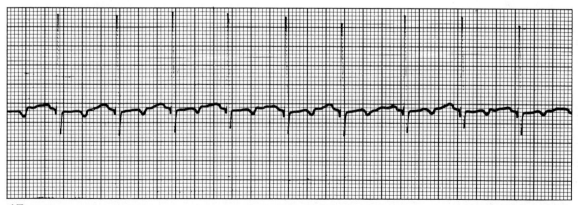

15

Practice ECG Answers

1. Sinus rhythm with AV dissociation with an accelerated junctional rhythm
2. Junctional escape rhythm
3. Sinus rhythm
4. Sinus rhythm with bundle branch block and AV dissociation with an accelerated junctional rhythm
5. Atrial flutter with 2:1 conduction
6. Junctional escape rhythm
7. Supraventricular tachycardia
8. Accelerated junctional rhythm
9. Sinus arrhythmia
10. Atrial fibrillation
11. Sinus arrhythmia with AV dissociation with an accelerated junctional rhythm
12. Junctional tachycardia
13. Sinus tachycardia with first degree AV block
14. Sinus rhythm with AV dissociation with an accelerated junctional rhythm
15. Sinus tachycardia

6

VENTRICULAR RHYTHMS

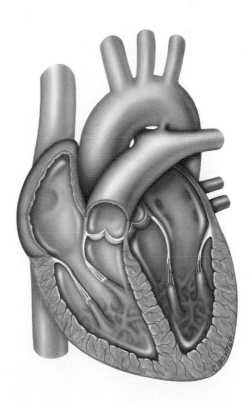

VENTRICULAR RHYTHMS

Ventricular Escape Rhythm

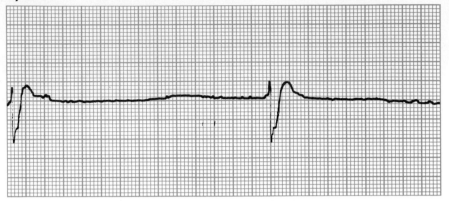

CRITERIA

1. 4-6 or more ventricular escape beats in a row at a regular rate below 40/min.

2. QRS complexes are wide and bizarre (.12 second or greater)

3. No ectopic P waves are present

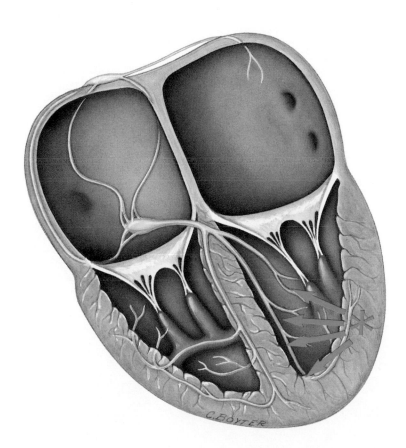

VENTRICULAR RHYTHMS

Accelerated Ventricular Rhythm

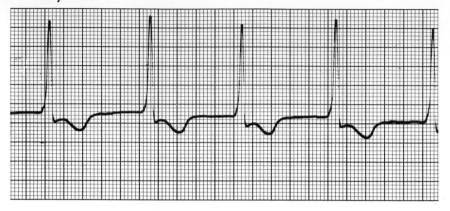

CRITERIA

1. **4-6 or more ventricular ectopic beats in a row at a regular rate between 40-100/min.**

2. **QRS complexes are wide and bizarre (.12 second or greater)**

3. **No ectopic P waves are present**

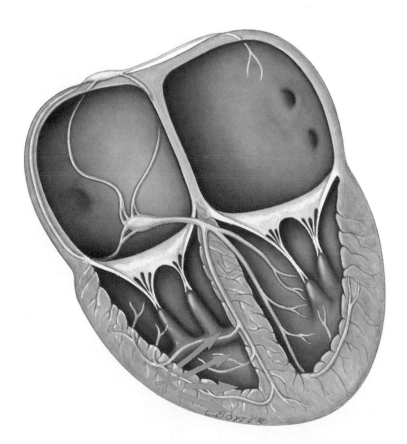

VENTRICULAR RHYTHMS

Ventricular Tachycardia

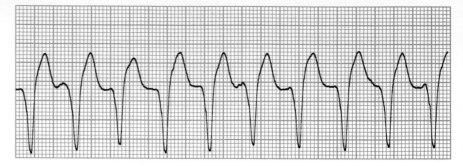

DIFFERENTIAL DIAGNOSIS OF ARRHYTHMIAS

CRITERIA

1. **4-6 or more VPCs in a row at a regular rate over 100/min.**

2. **QRS complexes are wide and bizarre (.12 second or greater)**

3. **No ectopic P waves are present**

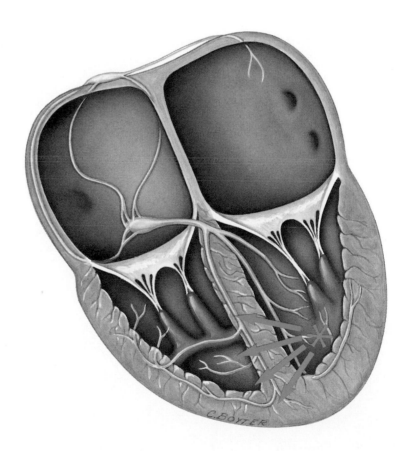

VENTRICULAR RHYTHMS

Ventricular Flutter

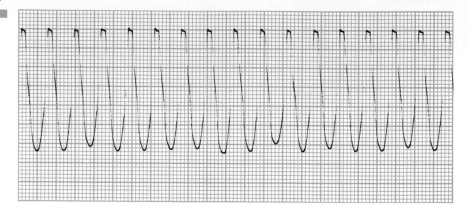

DIFFERENTIAL DIAGNOSIS OF ARRHYTHMIAS

CRITERIA

1. One or more ectopic foci in the ventricles fires at a regular rate between 150-300/min.

2. No atrial activity is present and the QRS complexes appear to merge into one another with no visible ST segments or T waves

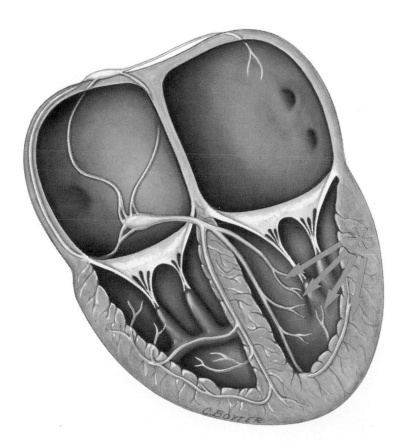

VENTRICULAR RHYTHMS

Ventricular Fibrillation

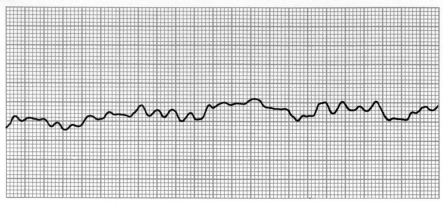

DIFFERENTIAL DIAGNOSIS OF ARRHYTHMIAS

CRITERIA

1. Multifocal ventricular ectopic foci fire at a rate between 150-500/min. with a chaotic rhythm

2. No atrial activity or QRS complexes and associated ST-T waves are present

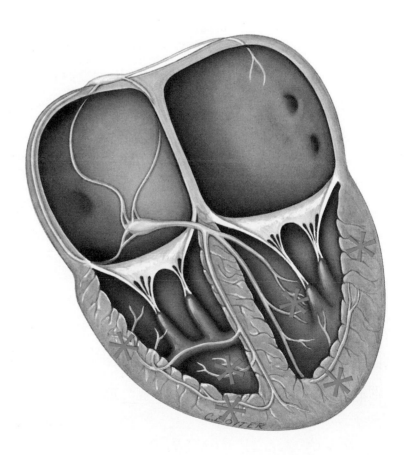

Ventricular rhythms originate in an area in the ventricles and are composed of 4-6 or more wide (.12 second or greater) and bizarre ectopic beats in a row. There are no associated ectopic P waves with ventricular rhythms. They are categorized by rate and configuration. The rapid depolarizations and contractions that take place during ventricular tachycardia, ventricular flutter, and ventricular fibrillation compromise the systemic circulation and are an emergency situation.

During ventricular escape rhythms, accelerated ventricular rhythms and ventricular tachycardias, it is the foci in the ventricles that are firing and causing ventricular depolarizations. Normally, the depolarization wave does not travel retrogradely to the atria, so if the atria are in sinus rhythm the sinus P wave is unaffected by the ventricular rhythm and continues on uninterrupted. These two rhythms occur simultaneously, temporarily unaffected by each other, and demonstrate AV dissociation. When this occurs, the sinus P wave occurs regularly, superimposing itself on top of or hidden within the QRS complexes, ST segments, and T waves. Occasionally, one of the sinus P waves falls outside the refractory period of the heart and is able to conduct its impulse down to the ventricles through normal conduction pathways and produce a QRS from the sinus rhythm in the midst of the ectopic ventricular rhythm. This is called a **ventricular capture beat**—the ventricles are "captured" by the sinus impulse.

Ventricular Escape Rhythm

Is a run of 4-6 or more ventricular escape beats in a row at a regular rate below 40 beats per minute. If long ventricular pauses occur the first line of defense are AV junctional escape rhythms. If the AV junction can't be motivated to respond to the slow heart rate, the ventricles react with a ventricular escape rhythm. Ventricular escape rhythms are commonly seen during complete AV block.

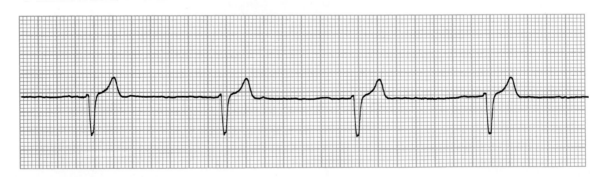

Ventricular escape rhythm.

Accelerated Ventricular Rhythm

Is a run of 4-6 or more ventricular ectopic beats in a row at a regular rate between 40-100 beats per minute. It is a much more benign arrhythmia than the slow ventricular rates of a ventricular escape rhythm associated with complete heart block and the rapid ventricular rates with ventricular tachycardia.

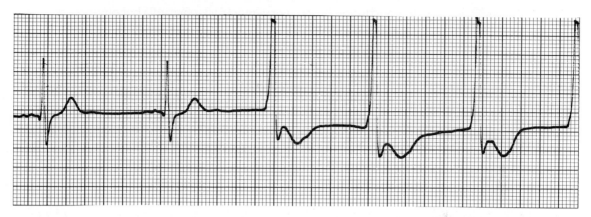

Sinus bradycardia and a run of accelerated ventricular rhythm.

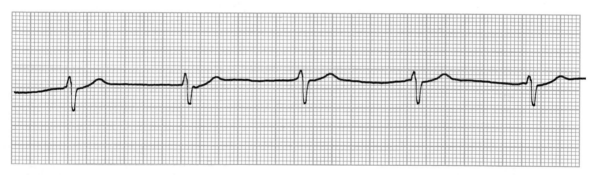

Accelerated ventricular rhythm.

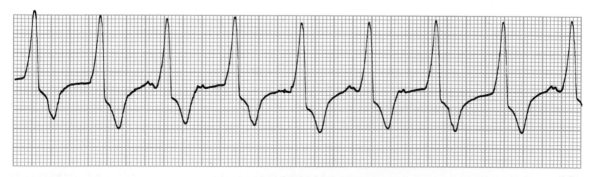

Accelerated ventricular rhythm with AV dissociation and sinus tachycardia at 110 beats per minute.

Ventricular Tachycardia

Is a run of 4-6 or more VPCs in a row at a regular rate over 100 beats per minute. If the tachycardia is multifocal in origin the rate will be irregular.

The diagnosis of ventricular tachycardia would be clear cut if it weren't for supraventricular tachycardias with bundle branch block or with aberration. (Refer to Chapter 7) Identification of sinus P waves displaying AV dissociation and fusion beats favor ventricular tachycardia but other possibilities still exist. This is a very serious arrhythmia and if not terminated often progresses to ventricular flutter and fibrillation.

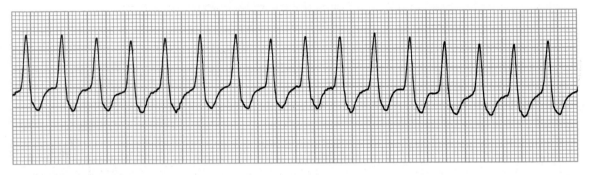

Ventricular tachycardia.

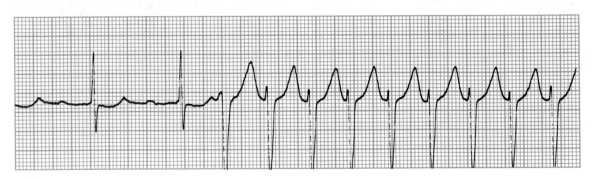

Sinus rhythm with first degree AV block with a run of ventricular tachycardia.

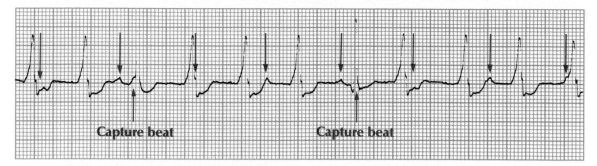

Ventricular tachycardia with AV dissociation and sinus rhythm and two capture beats. The sinus P waves are identified with arrows.

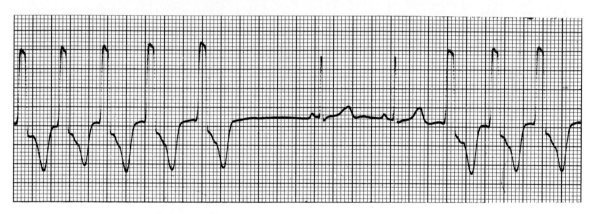

Sinus rhythm with two short bursts of ventricular tachycardia.

Ventricular Flutter

Is the rapid firing of one or more ectopic ventricular foci at a fairly regular rate over 150 beats per minute. No atrial activity is present. ST segments and T waves cannot be distinguished. If left untreated, ventricular flutter usually deteriorates into ventricular fibrillation.

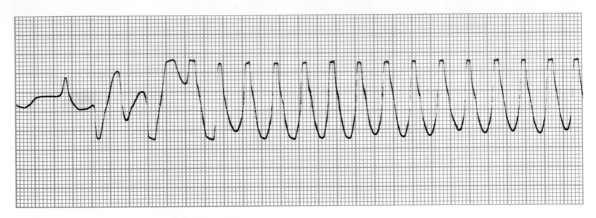

Multifocal ventricular tachycardia escalating into ventricular flutter.

Ventricular Fibrillation

Is the rapid firing of multifocal ectopic ventricular foci at a rate over 150 per minute with a chaotic rhythm. No atrial activity is present and there are no QRS complexes or associated ST-T waves. Ventricular fibrillation can appear as coarse, small, erratic configurations or as a fine, virtually flat line and is the most serious arrhythmia that can occur.

Interpretation confusion can only occur with the artifact created in the event of a loose electrode. No other arrhythmia mimics ventricular fibrillation.

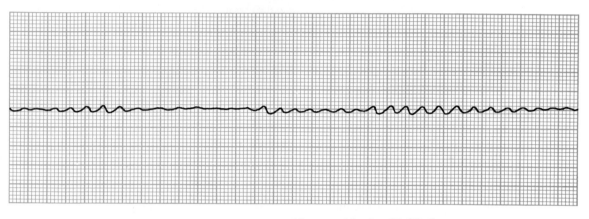

Fine ventricular fibrillation.

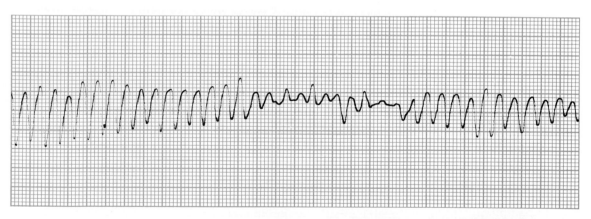

Ventricular flutter alternating with ventricular fibrillation.

Differential Diagnosis

During rapid sinus rates, when sinus P waves are more difficult to identify, the wide and bizarre QRS complexes associated with bundle branch block often mimic ventricular tachycardia. Sinus tachycardia with bundle branch block will maintain a constant PR interval for each QRS complex throughout the strip. Ventricular tachycardia displays no associated P waves.

Ventricular tachycardia with AV dissociation with the SA node might be diagnosed as sinus rhythm with bundle branch block because of the occurrence of sinus P waves at a regular rate. But there are no constant PR intervals and the sinus P waves bear no relationship with the QRS complexes, confirming the diagnosis of ventricular tachycardia.

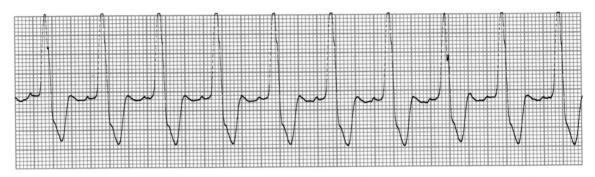

Sinus rhythm at 100 beats per minute with bundle branch block. The observation of sinus P waves with a constant PR interval preceding each QRS rules out ventricular tachycardia.

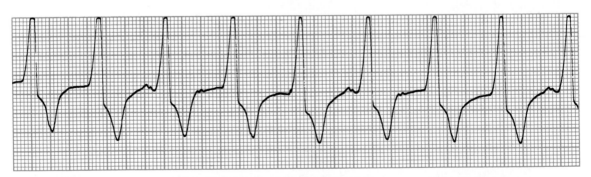

Sinus tachycardia with AV dissociation and accelerated ventricular rhythm. The sinus P waves bear no relationship to the QRS complexes but simply occur at a regular rate before, during, and after the QRS complexes.

When the ventricular response to atrial fibrillation is rapid and bundle branch block is present, the diagnosis is easily confused with ventricular tachycardia. The clue for proper identification are the irregular R-R cycles displayed by atrial fibrillation. R-R cycles tend to appear regular during fast ventricular rates but on careful observation the irregularly, irregular ventricular response can be discerned.

Ventricular tachycardia and junctional tachycardia with bundle branch block are indiscernible on an ECG and either interpretation would be correct. If previous ECGs are available and bundle branch block has been previously diagnosed, then junctional tachycardia with bundle branch block would be correct.

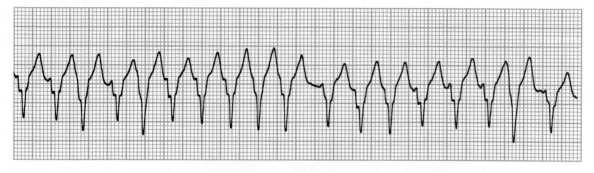

Atrial fibrillation with bundle branch block mimicking ventricular tachycardia. Notice the irregular R-R cycle compatible with atrial fibrillation.

PRACTICE ECGs

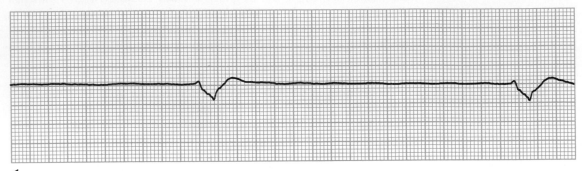

1

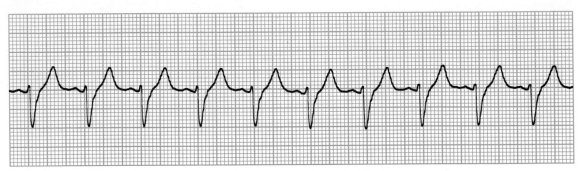

2

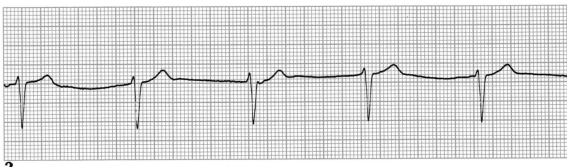

3

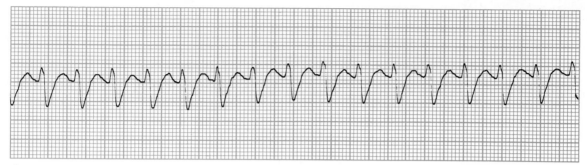

4

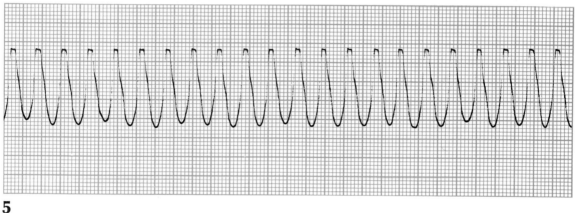

5

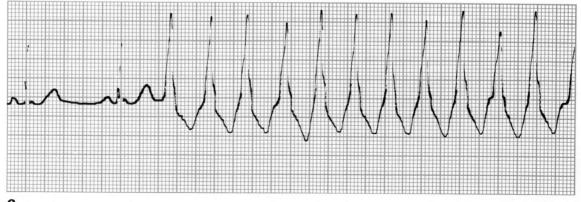

6

VENTRICULAR RHYTHMS

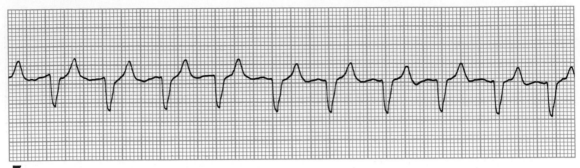

7

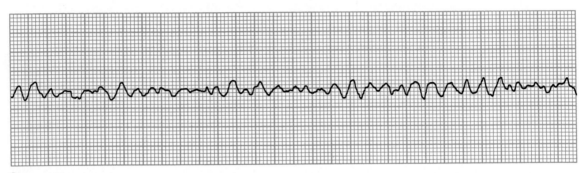

8

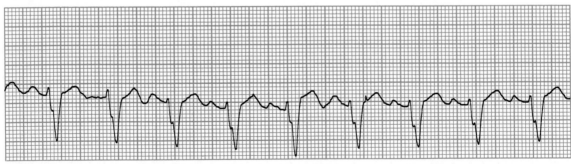

9

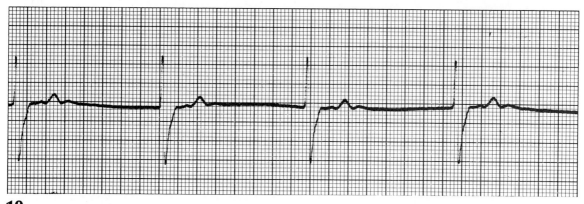

10

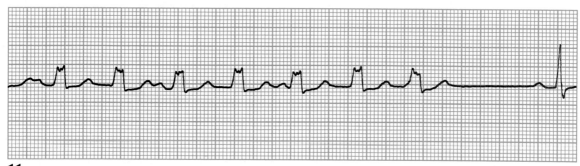

11

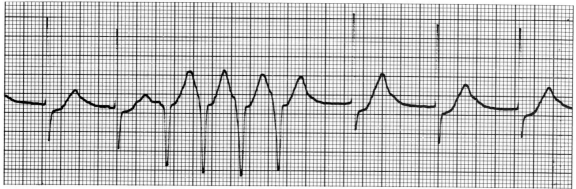

12

PRACTICE ECGs

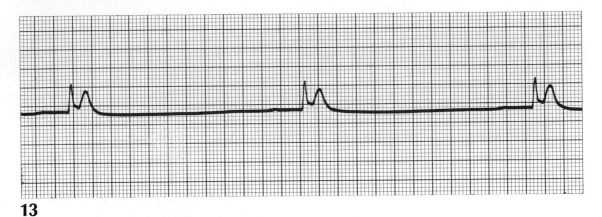

13

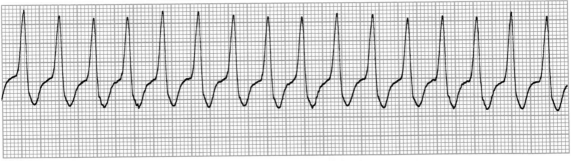

14

15

Practice ECG Answers

1. Ventricular escape rhythm
2. Sinus tachycardia with bundle branch block
3. Accelerated ventricular rhythm
4. Ventricular tachycardia
5. Ventricular flutter
6. Sinus rhythm with a burst of ventricular tachycardia
7. Accelerated ventricular rhythm
8. Ventricular fibrillation
9. Sinus rhythm with bundle branch block
10. Ventricular escape rhythm
11. Sinus rhythm with AV dissociation and an accelerated ventricular rhythm with a spontaneous conversion to sinus rhythm
12. Accelerated junctional rhythm with a short burst of ventricular tachycardia
13. Marked sinus bradycardia with first degree AV block and ST elevation
14. Atrial fibrillation with bundle branch block
15. Ventricular tachycardia

7

ABERRATION

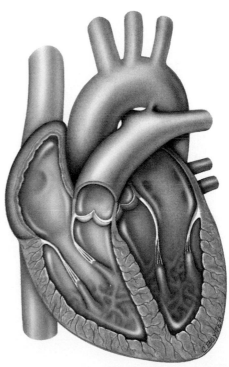

ABERRATION

APC with Aberration

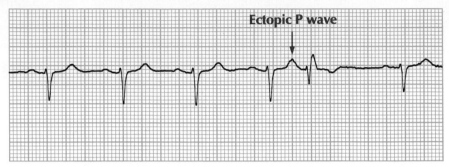

DIFFERENTIAL DIAGNOSIS OF ARRHYTHMIAS

CRITERIA

1. Upright, early ectopic P wave immediately followed by a bizarre and usually wide QRS complex

2. Noncompensatory pause following the APC.

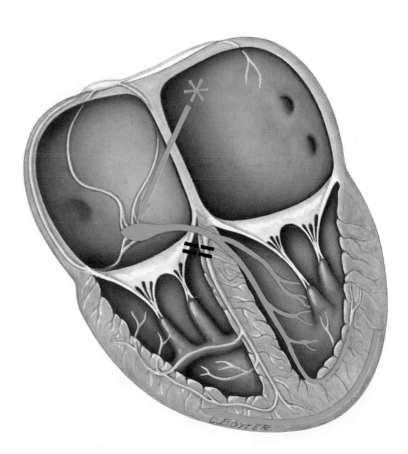

ABERRATION

JPC with Aberration

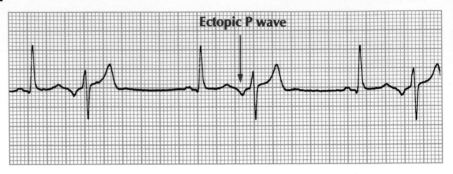

Ectopic P wave

CRITERIA

1. Inverted, early ectopic P wave either preceding or immediately following a bizarre
   and usually wide QRS complex.

2. Noncompensatory pause following the
   JPC.

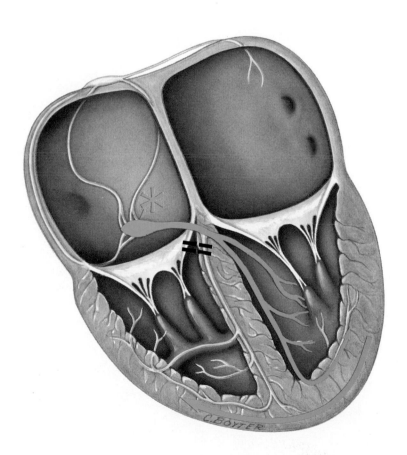

ABERRATION

ABERRATION

Atrial Fibrillation or Atrial Flutter with Aberration

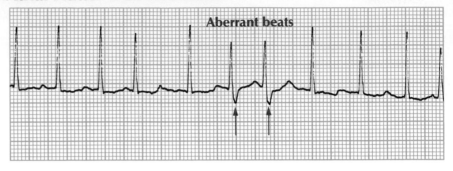

Aberrant beats

CRITERION

1. **Long R-R cycle followed closely by a bizarre and usually wide QRS complex favors aberration**

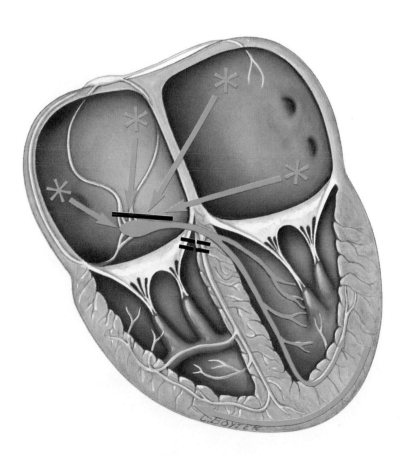

ABERRATION

Supraventricular Tachycardia with Aberration

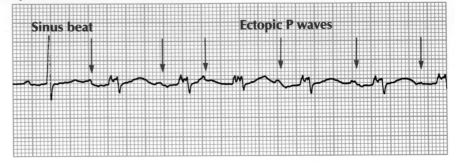

CRITERION

1. **Wide and bizarre QRS complexes occurring at a rapid rate each preceded or followed by an ectopic P wave superimposed on a T wave.**

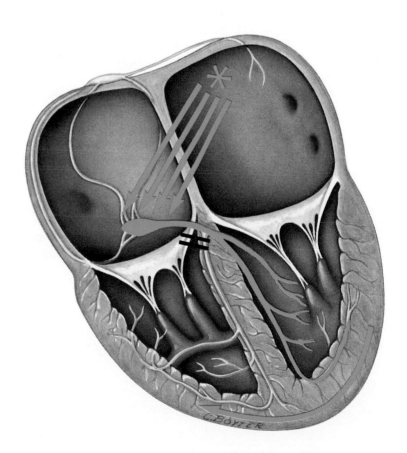

Aberration provides the greatest challenge in arrhythmia interpretation. Aberration is a variation from the normal QRS configuration, and it occurs when a sinus or supraventricular impulse finds one of the bundle branches to be refractory from the previous beat. The right bundle branch has a longer refractory period than either the left anterior or posterior fascicle and is generally the temporary inoperable conduction pathway. The configuration of the QRS complex with aberrant ventricular conduction therefore shows a right bundle branch pattern. Conduction takes place abnormally from one ventricle to the other through connections in the ventricular myocardium. Because of the abnormal direction and the subsequent delay in conduction, a bizarre and usually wide QRS complex results. Variations in degree of aberrancy depend on the amount of depolarization which follows normal conduction pathways and that which is conducted abnormally from one ventricle to the other.

Aberration can occur:

1. If an APC or JPC occurs very close to the previous QRS
2. During irregular rates found in atrial fibrillation and atrial flutter, when a long R-R cycle (when the refractory period of the bundle branches normally lengthens) is followed by a short R-R cycle (**Ashman Phenomena**)
3. During rapid supraventricular tachycardias

Aberration imitates VPCs and ventricular tachycardias but one must be able to make as accurate a diagnosis as possible in spite of the difficulty generated by the impersonation. To confirm the diagnosis of aberration with APCs and JPCs, look for the hidden ectopic P waves in the previous T waves, during atrial fibrillation and atrial flutter look for the long R-R cycle preceding the wide and bizarre looking QRS, and during rapid tachycardias search for ectopic P waves superimposed on top of the T waves. The initial portion of the QRS complex in an aberrantly conducted beat usually has the same direction as the normally conducted beat.

APCs and JPCs With Aberration

APCs and JPCs will demonstrate aberrancy if they occur so closely to the previous QRS complexes that they find one of the bundle branches still refractory and unable to conduct their impulse. Conduction will continue through the remaining bundle branch and with delay, through abnormal conduction pathways, depolarize the other ventricle. This gives rise to varying configurations in the QRS complexes preceded or followed by early, ectopic, upright or inverted P waves. The pauses following either APCs or JPCs will usually be noncompensatory.

Examine the T waves before the wide and bizarre QRS complexes for hidden ectopic, P waves. They often distort the previous T wave but can be found by careful examination.

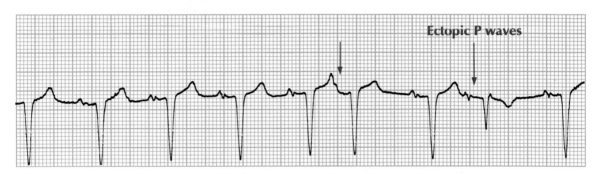

Sinus rhythm with two isolated APCs. The second APC is conducted with aberration. Notice the early ectopic P wave preceding the different looking QRS, confirming the diagnosis of APC with aberration.

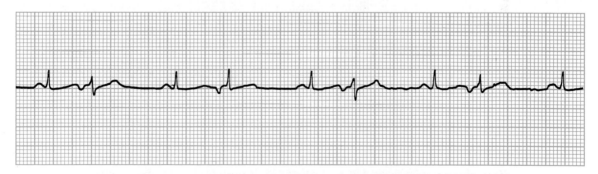

Sinus rhythm with JPCs in bigeminy showing various degrees of aberration.

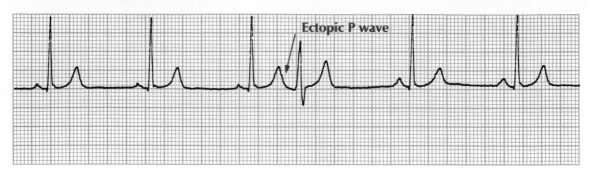

Sinus bradycardia with an APC with aberration. The ectopic P wave is
very subtly located on the downslope of the T wave.

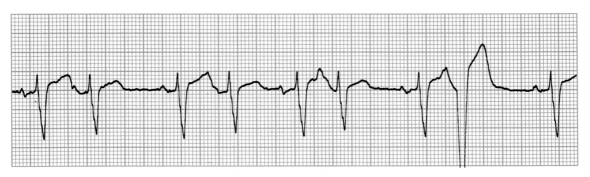

Sinus rhythm with bundle branch block and APCs in bigeminy.
The last APC displays aberration.

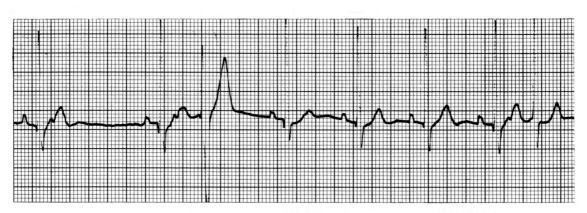

Sinus rhythm with three APCs. The first APC is nonconducted, the second
is conducted with aberration, and the third APC is conducted normally.

Atrial Fibrillation and Atrial Flutter with Aberration

During atrial fibrillation and atrial flutter the ventricular response varies and gives rise to both long and short R-R intervals. As the R-R cycle lengthens, so does the refractory period of the bundle branches. If a long R-R cycle is followed by a very short R-R cycle the next QRS is prone to display aberration. This type of aberrancy is termed the Ashman phenomenon.

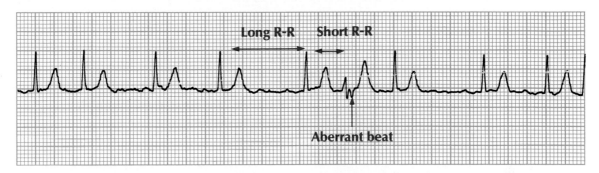

Atrial fibrillation with a long R-R cycle followed by a short R-R cycle favors aberration of the next QRS. (Ashman phenomena)

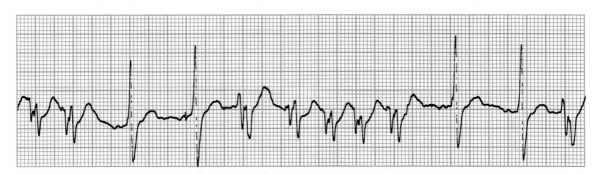

Atrial fibrillation with bundle branch block with bursts of aberrant beats.

Supraventricular Tachycardia with Aberration

During rapid supraventricular tachycardias one of the bundle branches is unable to repolarize quickly enough to conduct the rapid impulses and aberration occurs. Ectopic upright P waves either precede each QRS during atrial tachycardia or ectopic inverted P waves either precede or follow each QRS during junctional tachycardia. A careful inspection of the T waves and ST segments must be made to determine if ectopic P waves are present.

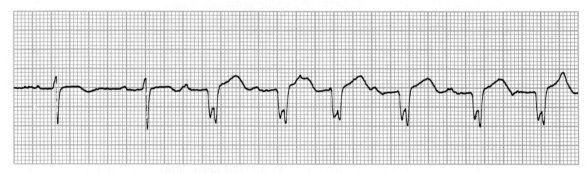

Sinus rhythm with first degree AV block with a run of atrial tachycardia with aberration. Ectopic P waves are clearly visible preceding each QRS.

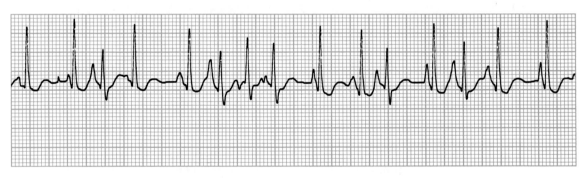

Multifocal atrial tachycardia with aberration during rapid rates.

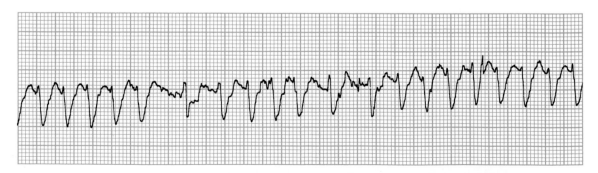

Supraventricular tachycardia with aberrancy.

Differential Diagnosis

Differentiating between supraventricular beats with aberration and ventricular beats can be mildly difficult at best and impossible at worst. The best clue in diagnosing aberrations is the early ectopic P wave—either upright or inverted. This cinches the diagnosis of aberration. A VPC will display no ectopic P waves, although the sinus P wave will sometimes be seen buried within the ST-T waves of the VPC or precede an end diastolic VPC.

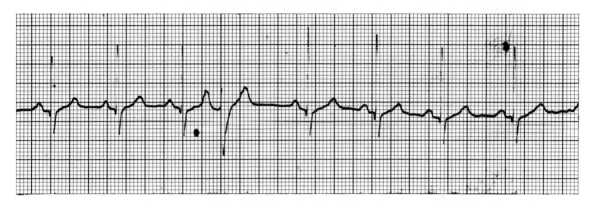

Sinus rhythm with an APC with aberration. The ectopic P wave can be seen distorting the T wave of the previous beat.

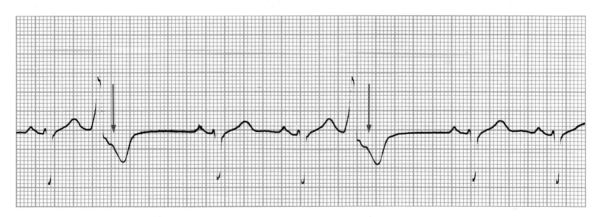

Sinus rhythm with two unifocal VPCs. There are no ectopic P waves preceding the wide and bizarre QRS complexes, ruling out the diagnosis of APCs or JPCs with aberration. Sinus P waves can be seen in the ST segment of each VPC and are identified with arrows.

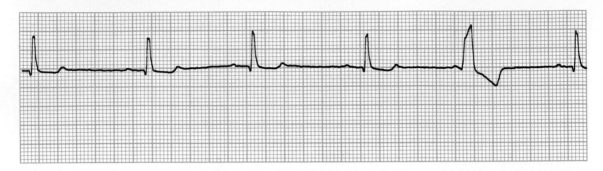

Sinus bradycardia with an end diastolic VPC. This is not an APC with aberration. The P wave preceding the wide and bizarre QRS complex is the sinus P wave arriving exactly on time and followed by a VPC.

If sinus rhythm with bundle branch block is the predominant rhythm and an APC fires—it will also conduct in a bundle branch block pattern. Even though the APC has a wide and bizarre QRS, this does not represent aberration, but rather the conduction disorder of bundle branch block.

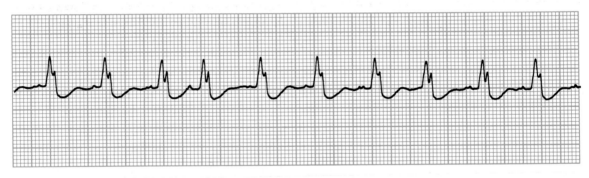

Sinus rhythm with bundle branch block and one APC.

Distinguishing VPCs from aberration during atrial fibrillation and atrial flutter offers more difficulty. The clues in this case are the long and short R-R sequences. If a wide and bizarre QRS follows a long R-R cycle very closely, this would favor aberration. If however, this same wide and bizarre QRS recurs following short R-R cycles and occurs far enough away from previous T waves so as not to interfere with the refractory periods of the bundle branches, it would favor a VPC. The occurrence of multifocal wide and bizarre QRS complexes suggests VPCs.

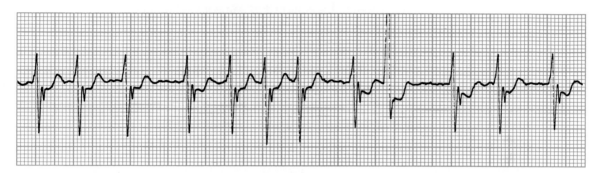

Atrial fibrillation with one aberrant beat. The wide and bizarre QRS complex is preceded by a long-short R-R cycle favoring aberration.

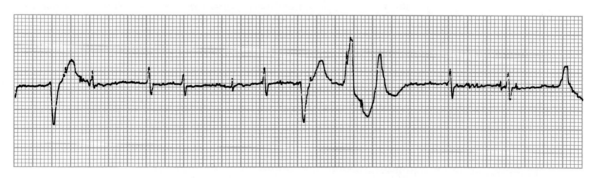

Atrial fibrillation with five multifocal VPCs with one episode of three in a row.

Supraventricular tachycardia with aberration versus ventricular tachycardia is the biggest problem and by far the most important challenge in arrhythmia interpretation. Unfortunately, it is often impossible to make a distinction between these two possibilities and you're left with an either/or interpretation. If you're lucky enough to catch the initial beat of the tachycardia it can solve the interpretation problem. Oftentimes tachycardias begin with a slower rate and if ectopic P waves are present they can be observed much easier than during faster rates. Even with rapid rates, ectopic P waves can sometimes be observed superimposed on top of previous T waves. Careful observation and some luck is required.

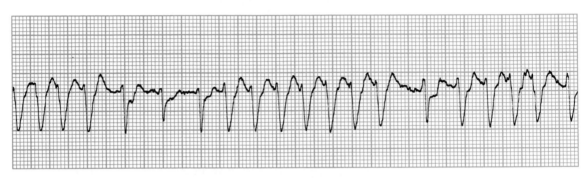

Supraventricular tachycardia with aberrancy. As the R-R cycle lengthens the QRS complex narrows, supporting the diagnosis of aberration.

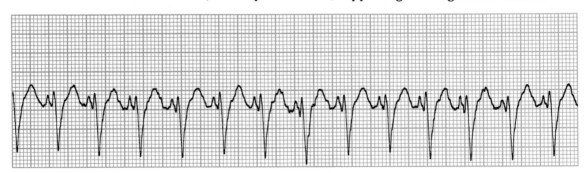

Supraventricular tachycardia with aberrancy. P waves are visible preceding each QRS with a constant PR interval ruling out a ventricular tachycardia.

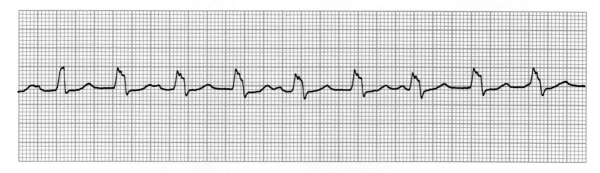

Accelerated ventricular rhythm. Sinus P waves can be seen occurring throughout the strip with varying PR intervals, demonstrating AV dissociation during a ventricular rhythm, ruling out a supraventricular tachycardia with aberrancy.

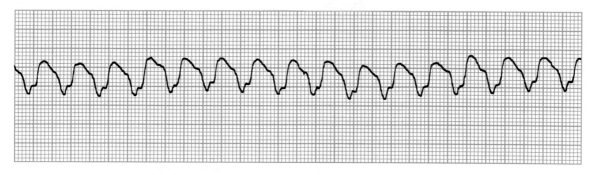

Ventricular tachycardia versus supraventricular tachycardia with aberration.

PRACTICE ECGs

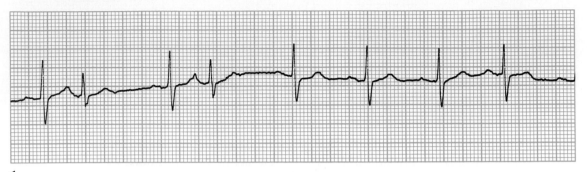

1

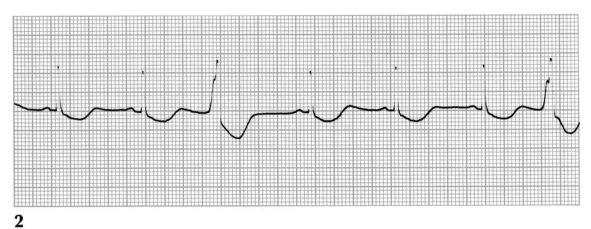

2

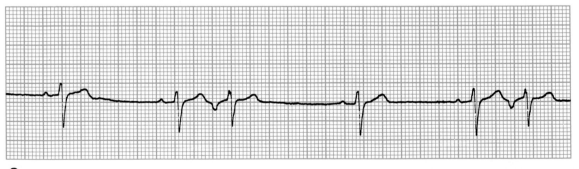

3

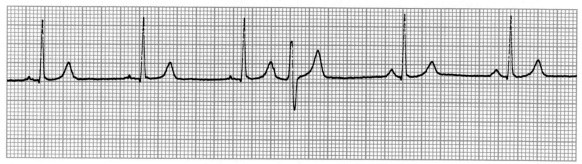

4

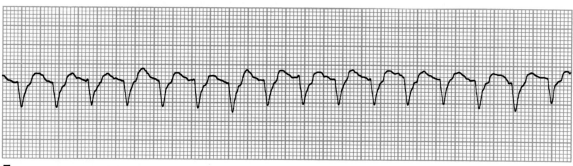

5

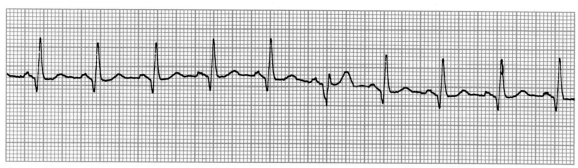

6

PRACTICE ECGs

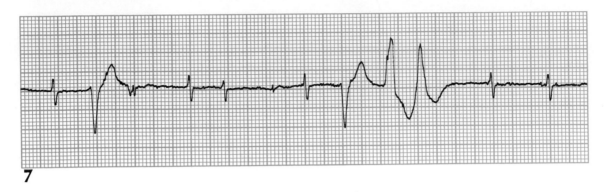

7

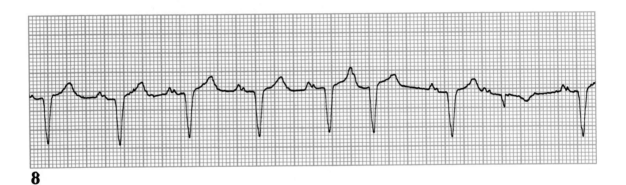

8

9

DIFFERENTIAL DIAGNOSIS OF ARRHYTHMIAS

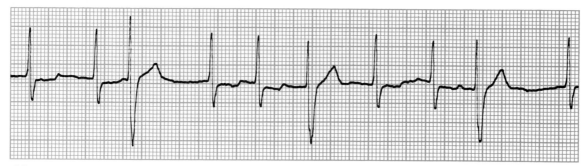

10

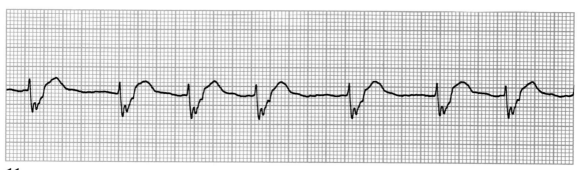

11

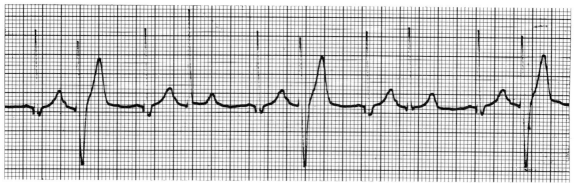

12

PRACTICE ECGs

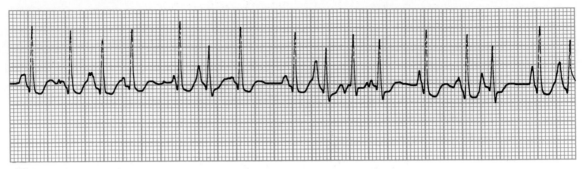

13

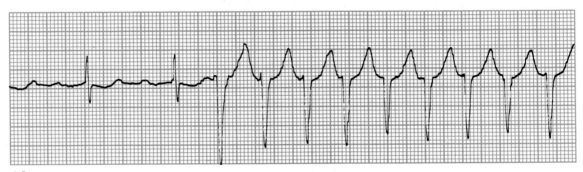

14

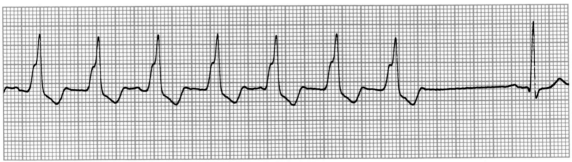

15

Practice ECG Answers

1. Sinus rhythm with two APCs with aberration
2. Sinus rhythm with two unifocal VPCs
3. Sinus bradycardia with two JPCs with aberration
4. Sinus bradycardia with one APC with aberration
5. Ventricular tachycardia versus supraventricular tachycardia with aberration
6. Sinus rhythm with one end diastolic VPC
7. Atrial fibrillation with four multifocal VPCs
8. Sinus rhythm with two isolated APCs, the second APC is conducted with aberration
9. Sinus rhythm with two isolated APCs, the second APC is conducted with aberration
10. Atrial fibrillation with aberrant beats
11. Atrial fibrillation with bundle branch block
12. Sinus rhythm with APCs in bigeminy, every other APC is conducted with aberration
13. Multifocal atrial tachycardia, some beats conducted with aberration
14. Sinus rhythm with first degree AV block with a burst of ventricular tachycardia
15. Ventricular tachycardia with AV dissociation and sinus rhythm

8

AV BLOCK

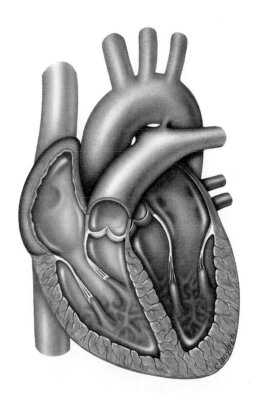

AV BLOCK

2nd Degree AV Block Wenckebach

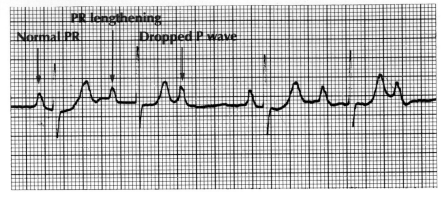

DIFFERENTIAL DIAGNOSIS OF ARRHYTHMIAS

CRITERIA

1. **P-P cycle is regular and the PR interval progressively lengthens from one QRS to another until a P wave is not conducted to the ventricles (dropped P wave) and a ventricular pause occurs**

2. **QRS resembles that of the regular cardiac rhythm**

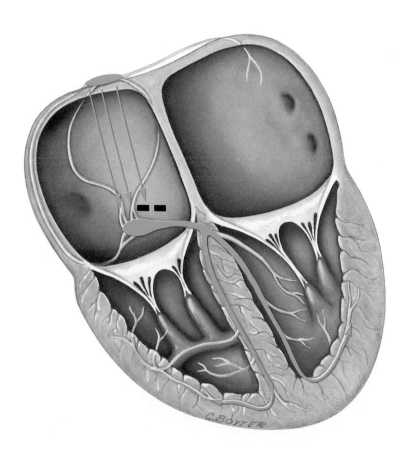

AV BLOCK

AV BLOCK

2nd Degree AV Block Mobitz

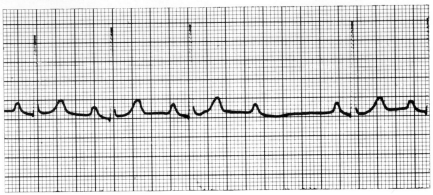

CRITERIA

1. **PR interval remains constant and P-P cycle is regular until a sinus P wave is dropped and ventricular pause occurs**

2. **No more than one P wave in a row is dropped**

3. **QRS resembles that of the regular cardiac rhythm**

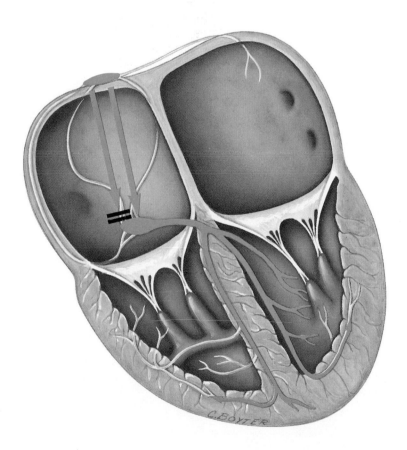

AV BLOCK

High Grade AV Block in Sinus Rhythm

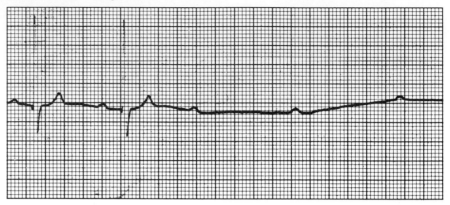

CRITERIA

1. **PR interval remains constant and P-P cycle is regular until two or more dropped P waves in a row occur producing long ventricular pauses**

2. **QRS resembles that of the regular cardiac rhythm**

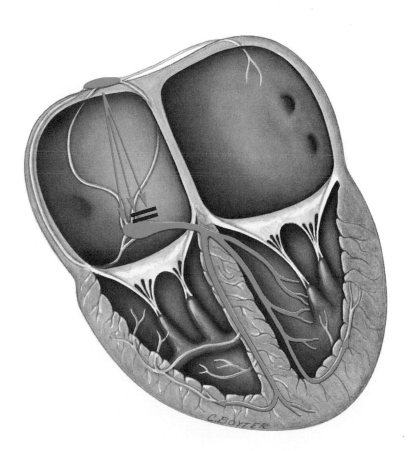

AV BLOCK

High Grade AV Block in Atrial Fibrillation and Flutter

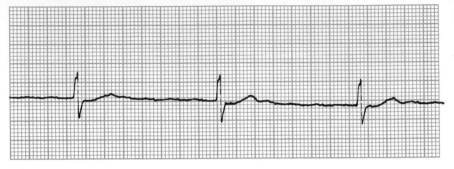

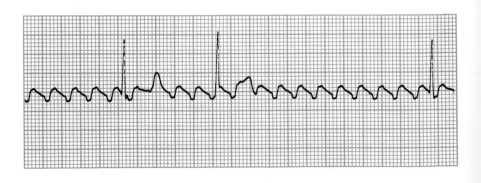

CRITERIA

1. Long ventricular pauses occur during atrial fibrillation and flutter

2. QRS resembles that of the regular cardiac rhythm

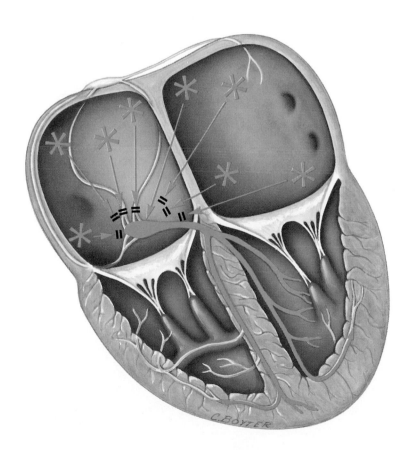

AV BLOCK

Complete AV Block

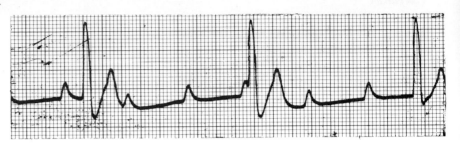

CRITERIA

1. No conduction occurs between the atria and ventricles

2. The atria are controlled by either sinus rhythm or an ectopic atrial focus and the ventricles are controlled by an ectopic junctional or ventricular escape rhythm

3. If the atria are in sinus rhythm, the P-P cycle will be regular but bear no relationship to the QRS complexes producing varying PR intervals

4. If the atria are fibrillating, the ventricular response will be uncharacteristically regular

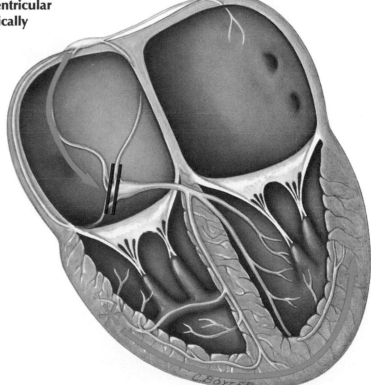

AV block is a delay or blockage of supraventricular impulses to the ventricles caused by a prolongation of the refractory period in the AV node or bundle branches. AV block is characterized by ventricular pauses and/or slow ventricular rates.

First Degree AV Block

First degree AV block is the lengthening of conduction time from the AV node to the ventricles and is characterized by a PR interval greater than .20 second.

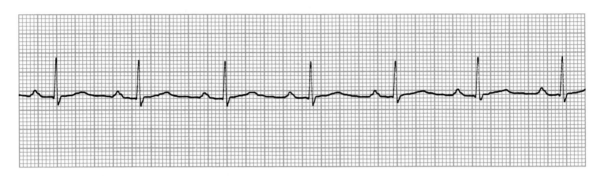

Sinus rhythm with first degree AV block.

Second Degree AV Block Wenckebach

Sinus P waves find it increasingly difficult to conduct their impulses to the ventricles due to prolongation of the refractory period in the AV node. PR intervals lengthen from one QRS to another, until conduction is prevented and a P wave occurs with no QRS complex following it. (**Dropped P wave**) During the ventricular pause the AV node recovers and the next P wave is conducted with its normal PR interval or slightly shorter. Generally, the blockage in the conduction system is in the AV node.

The pattern of PR lengthening followed by a dropped P wave represents a Wenckebach sequence. It begins with a normal PR interval and ends with the dropped P wave. A 3:2 sequence represents three P waves and two QRS complexes. The first PR interval would be normal, the second would demonstrate PR lengthening, and the third P wave would be the dropped P wave with no QRS following it.

Wenckebach can be an isolated event or can occur frequently with various sequences (2:1, 3:2, 4:3, 5:4, and so on). This is a benign arrhythmia and usually transient and if often associated with first degree AV block.

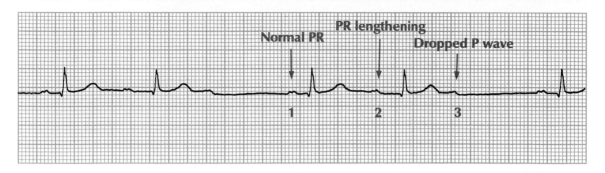

Sinus rhythm with first degree AV block with two episodes of 3:2
second degree AV block Wenckebach.

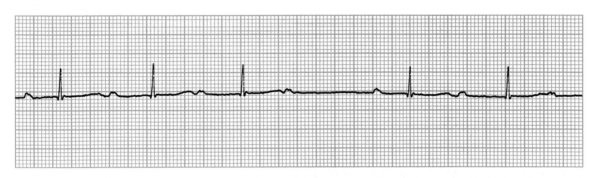

Sinus rhythm with first degree AV block and second degree AV block
Wenckebach with 4:3 and 3:2 sequences.

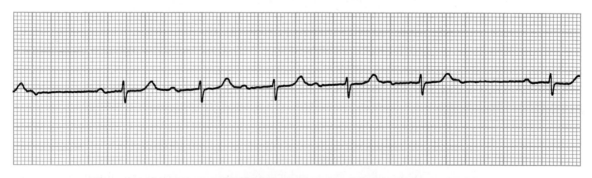

Sinus rhythm with first degree AV block and second degree AV block
Wenckebach with a 6:5 sequence.

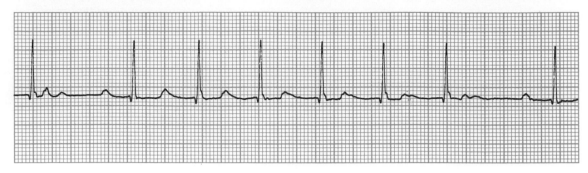

Sinus rhythm with first degree AV block and second degree AV block Wenckebach with a 7:6 sequence. Except for the first P wave of the Wenckebach cycle, all the sinus P waves are buried in the T waves of the previous beats.

During a 2:1 Wenckebach sequence there is no time for the PR interval to lengthen. The first PR is normal and the second P wave is dropped.

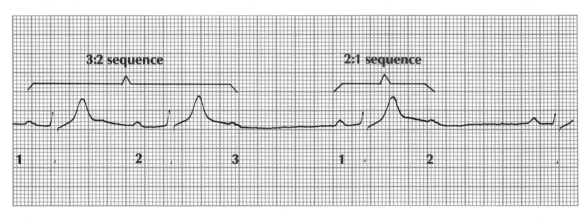

Sinus rhythm with first degree AV block and second degree AV block Wenckebach with a 3:2 and 2:1 sequence.

Second Degree AV Block Mobitz

In sinus rhythm, P waves occur regularly, PR intervals are constant and without any warning a P wave is dropped and a ventricular pause occurs. This is due to a intermittent prolongation of the refractory period usually distal to the bundle of His, in one of the bundle branches. The ventricular pause allows the conduction system to recover and the next P wave is conducted normally. P waves are dropped intermittently, but never more than one in a row.

DIFFERENTIAL DIAGNOSIS OF ARRHYTHMIAS

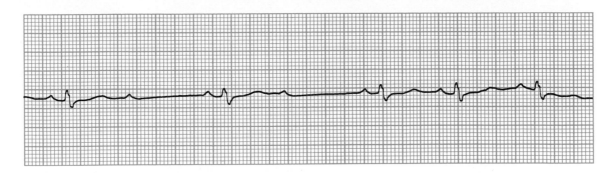

Sinus rhythm with two episodes of second degree AV block Mobitz.

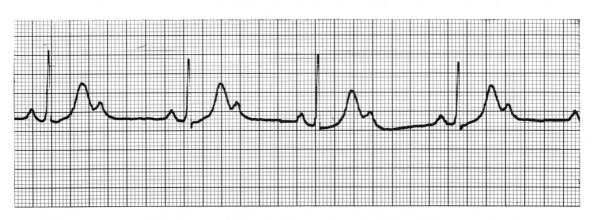

Sinus rhythm with second degree AV block Mobitz.

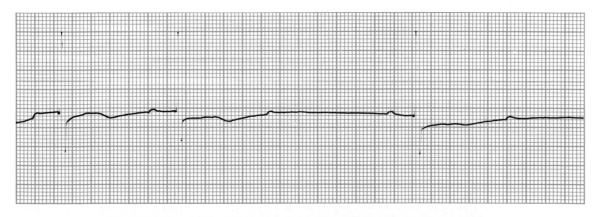

Sinus bradycardia with first degree AV block with 2 episodes of second degree AV block Mobitz.

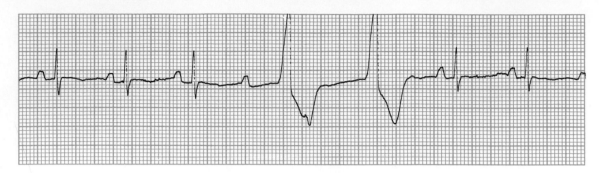

**Sinus rhythm with one episode of second degree AV block Mobitz with
two ventricular escape beats terminating the pause.**

Second degree AV block Wenckebach with a 2:1 sequence, which displays
no PR lengthening before the dropped P wave, is unable to be distinguished
from second degree AV block Mobitz on a short rhythm strip. It is hoped
that if Wenckebach is the arrhythmia present other conduction sequences
(3:2, 4:3, etc.) will occur on longer rhythm strips and verify the diagnosis.

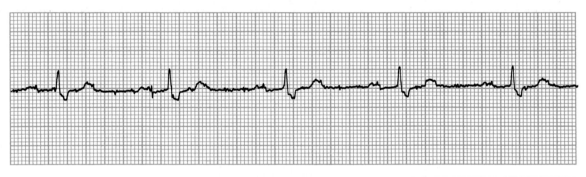

**Sinus rhythm with first degree AV block and bundle branch block with
2:1 second degree AV block either Mobitz or Wenckebach.**

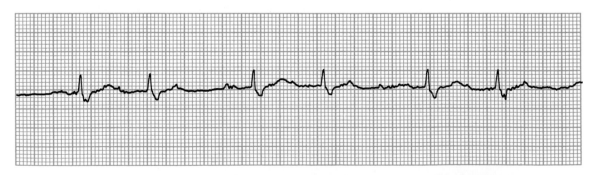

**This is the same patient as the previous ECG strip.
A 3:2 sequence is demonstrated, confirming the diagnosis of
second degree AV block Wenckebach.**

High Grade AV Block

In sinus rhythm, P waves occur regularly, PR intervals are of a constant duration, and more than one P wave in a row is dropped. This is due to a marked prolongation of the refractory period in the AV node or bundle branches.

In atrial fibrillation or atrial flutter, the presence of high grade block is suggested by long ventricular pauses or escape rhythms.

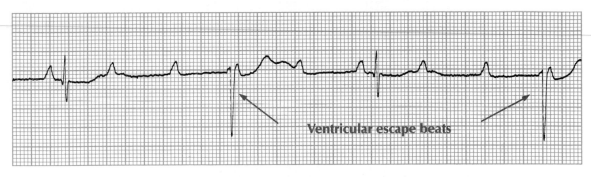

Sinus rhythm with high grade AV block and two ventricular escape beats terminating the ventricular pauses.

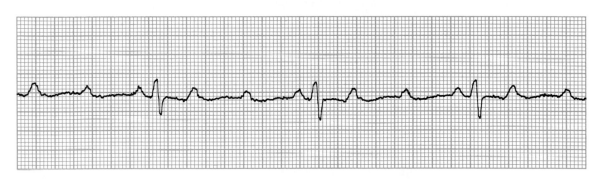

Sinus tachycardia with bundle branch block and high grade AV block.

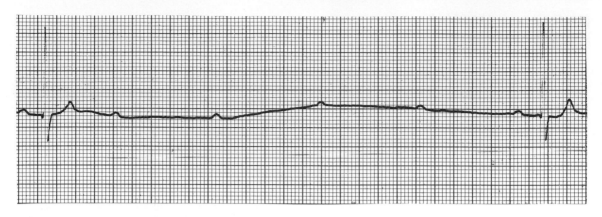

Sinus bradycardia with first degree AV block and high grade AV block.

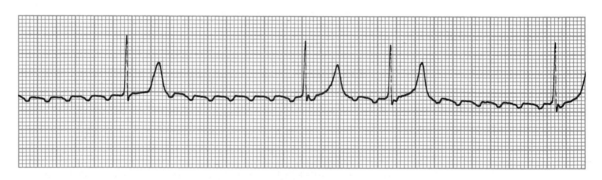

Atrial flutter with high grade AV block.

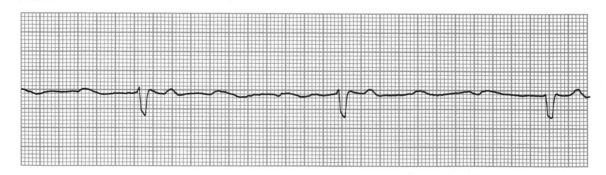

Atrial fibrillation with high grade AV block.

Complete AV Block

Third degree or complete AV block represents the most serious form of AV block. There is no conduction between the atria and the ventricles—each is under the control of separate pacemaking foci. The ventricles are controlled by either a junctional or ventricular escape rhythm and slow, regular ventricular rates occur.

If the atria are in sinus rhythm, the P-P cycle will be regular but bear no relationship to the QRS complexes producing varying PR intervals. The atrial rate is usually much faster than the escape rhythm which controls the ventricles. If the atria are fibrillating, none of the fibrillatory waves will be conducted to the ventricles and the usually irregular ventricular response will become uncharacteristically regular as the ventricles are controlled by an escape rhythm.

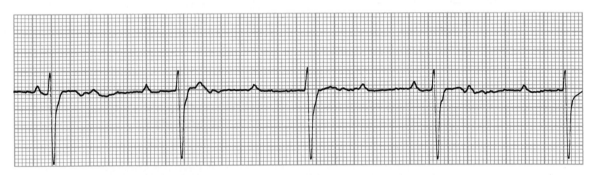

Sinus tachycardia with complete AV block and an accelerated ventricular rhythm.

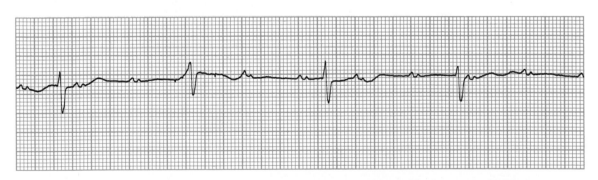

Sinus tachycardia with complete AV block and a junctional escape rhythm.

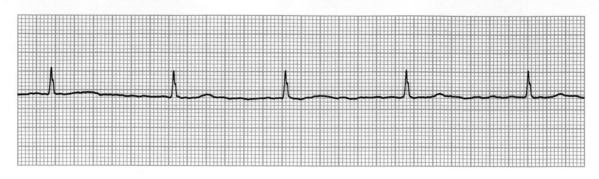

Atrial fibrillation with complete AV block and a junctional escape rhythm.

Differential Diagnosis

With prolonged first degree AV block the sinus P wave moves far enough leftward, away from the QRS complex, to lead one to diagnose a junctional rhythm. Careful observation reveals the presence of the P wave either superimposed on top of the previous T wave or occurring directly after it.

The ventricular pause and the dropped P wave that occurs with AV Wenckebach are similar to the criteria for nonconducted APCs. The important difference is that the nonconducted APC is an early P wave with a different configuration than that of the sinus P wave and with AV Wenckebach the P-P cycle is regular and the P waves all have the same configuration.

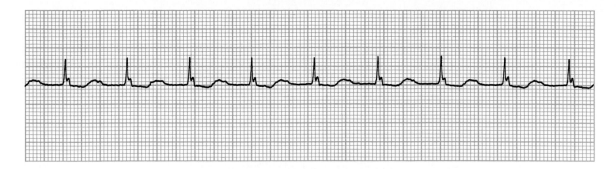

Sinus rhythm with marked first degree AV block. The sinus P waves can be seen superimposed on top of the T waves.

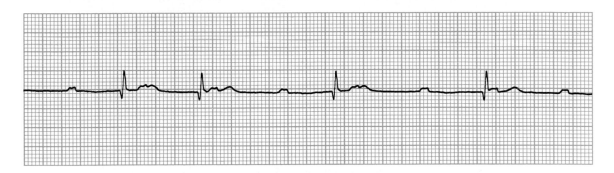

Sinus rhythm with marked first degree AV block and second degree AV block Wenckebach with 3:2 and 2:1 sequences. Because the P waves are buried in the T waves one might assume that they are early ectopic P waves, but they are sinus P waves with a regular P-P cycle.

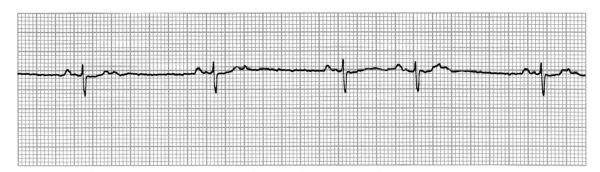

Sinus rhythm with four nonconducted APCs in bigeminy. The ectopic P waves superimposed on the T waves are clearly early beats and are not part of the regular sinus P wave cycle.

The varying PR interval associated with AV block Wenckebach can be confused with the varying PR interval in complete AV block. But the ventricular response in second degree AV Wenckebach demonstrates a pattern of shortening R-R cycles before a ventricular pause whereas in complete AV block the R-R cycle is regular and very slow as the ventricles are controlled by an escape rhythm.

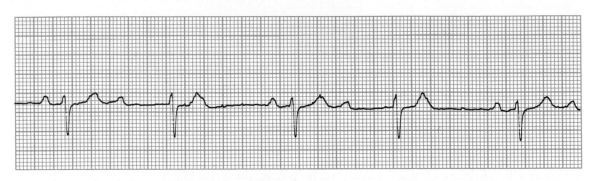

Sinus rhythm with first degree AV block and second degree AV block Wenckebach with 3:2 sequences. The R-R cycle shortens and the PR lengthens before the dropped P wave and ventricular pause.

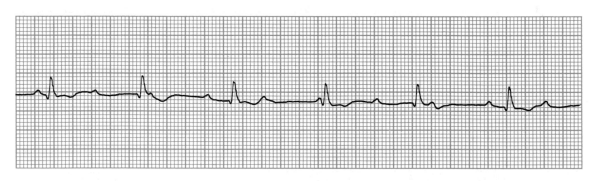

Sinus rhythm with complete AV block and an accelerated ventricular rhythm.

With AV dissociation there are dual rhythms occurring simultaneously in the heart—one focus controlling the atria and a second controlling the ventricles. But this arrhythmia is a temporary conduction disorder in which either the atrial or ventricle rate are nearly identical or the ventricular rate is rapid. In complete AV block there is a permanent lack of conduction between the atria and ventricles and each are controlled by separate pacemaking foci. The ventricular rates are substantially slower than the atrial rates and escape rhythms rescue the heart.

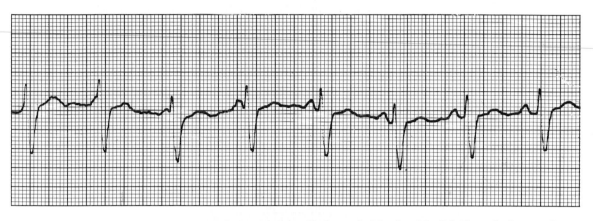

Sinus rhythm with bundle branch block with AV dissociation and an accelerated junctional rhythm. The atrial and ventricular rates are almost identical and the sinus P wave floats into and out of the QRS complexes. The last four beats are conducted normally.

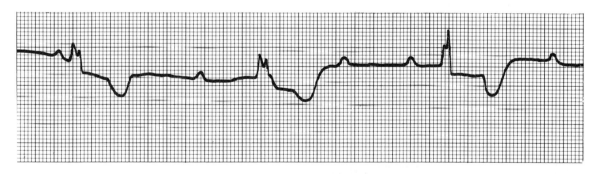

Sinus rhythm with complete AV block and a ventricular escape rhythm. Both the atrial and ventricular cycles are regular but the ventricular rate is much slower than the atrial rate as they are controlled by an escape rhythm.

PRACTICE ECGs

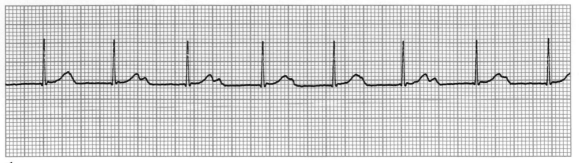

1

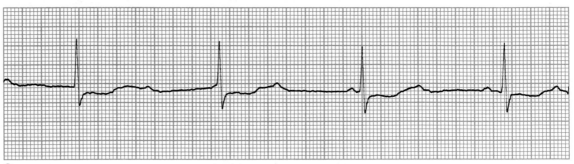

2

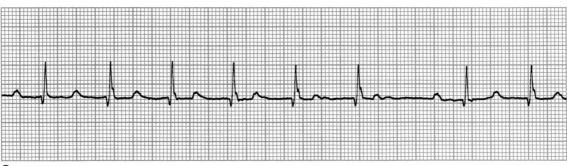

3

DIFFERENTIAL DIAGNOSIS OF ARRHYTHMIAS

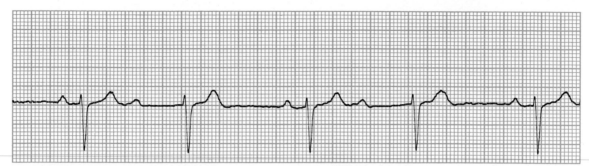

4

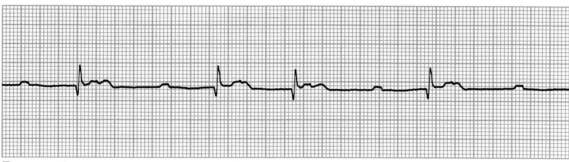

5

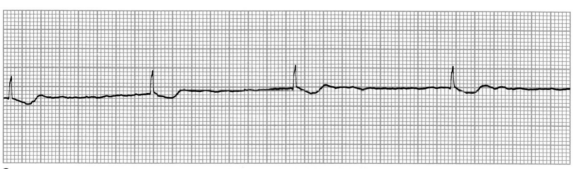

6

PRACTICE ECGs

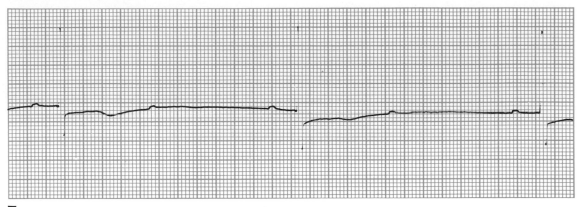

7

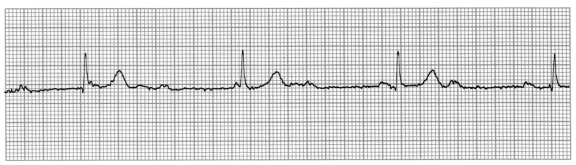

8

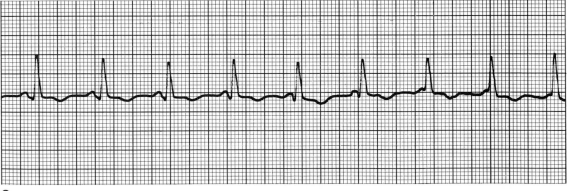

9

DIFFERENTIAL DIAGNOSIS OF ARRHYTHMIAS

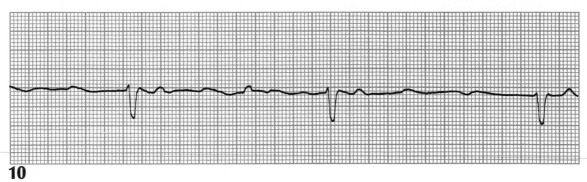

10

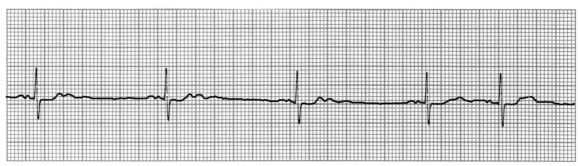

11

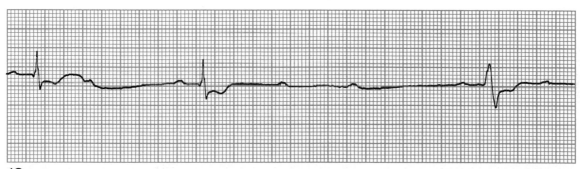

12

PRACTICE ECGs

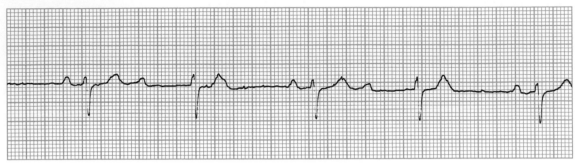

13

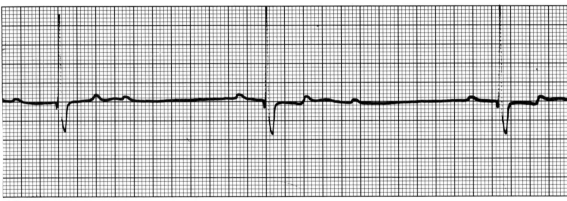

14

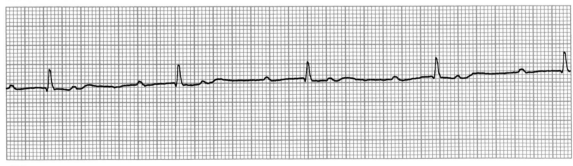

15

Practice ECG Answers

1. Sinus rhythm with first degree AV block
2. Sinus rhythm with complete heart block and a junctional escape rhythm
3. Sinus rhythm with first degree AV block and second degree AV block Wenckebach with a 7:6 sequence
4. Sinus rhythm with first degree AV block and second degree AV block Wenckebach with a 3:2 sequence
5. Sinus rhythm with first degree AV block and second degree AV block Wenckebach with 2:1 and 3:2 sequences
6. Atrial fibrillation with high grade AV block
7. Sinus bradycardia with first degree AV block and second degree AV block Mobitz
8. Sinus rhythm with complete heart block and a junctional escape rhythm
9. Sinus rhythm with AV dissociation and an accelerated junctional rhythm
10. Atrial fibrillation with bundle branch block and high grade AV block
11. Sinus rhythm with three nonconducted APCs in bigeminy
12. Sinus arrhythmia with first degree AV block and second degree AV block Mobitz and high grade AV block and a ventricular escape beat terminating a pause
13. Sinus rhythm with first degree AV block and second degree AV block Wenckebach with 3:2 sequences
14. Sinus bradycardia with first degree AV block and second degree AV block Mobitz
15. Sinus rhythm with first degree AV block and second degree AV block Mobitz

9

SA BLOCK

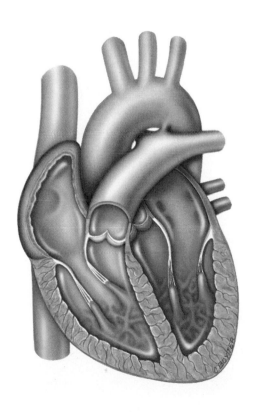

SA BLOCK

2nd Degree SA Block Wenckebach

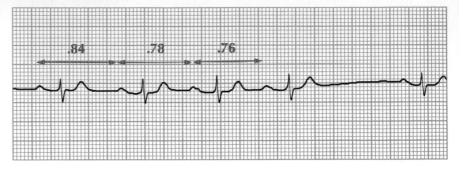

CRITERIA

1. **P-P cycle becomes progressively shorter until a ventricular pause occurs. No P waves or QRS complexes occur during the pause**

2. **The pause is less than twice the preceding P-P cycle**

3. **QRS resembles that of the regular cardiac rhythm**

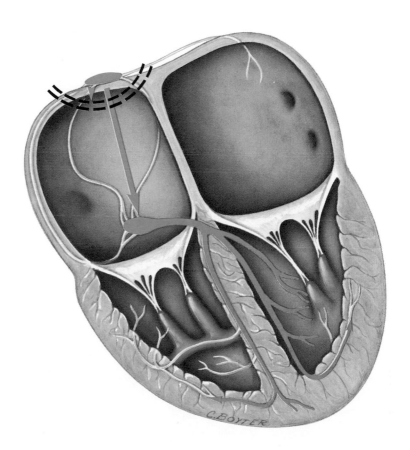

SA BLOCK

2nd Degree SA Block Mobitz

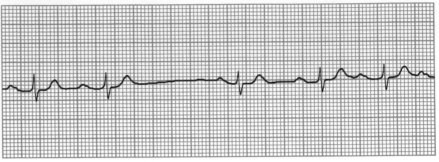

DIFFERENTIAL DIAGNOSIS OF ARRHYTHMIAS

CRITERIA

1. **The P-P cycle is constant before a ventricular pause occurs. No P waves or QRS complexes occur during the pause**

2. **The ventricular pause measures two or more times the length of the P-P cycle**

3. **QRS resembles that of the regular cardiac rhythm**

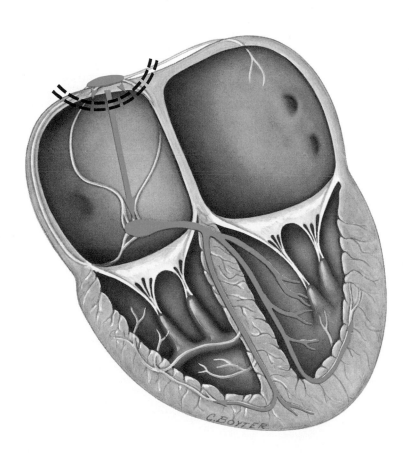

SA block is the delay or blockage of sinus impulses to the surrounding atrial musculature. The delay of sinus node impulses to the atria are not recorded on an ECG but blocked SA nodal impulses are displayed as the absence of P waves accompanied by ventricular pauses. In AV block, the delay or blockage occurs at the AV node or in the bundle branches so P waves are recorded but QRS complexes are missing. In SA block, the delay or blockage occurs between the SA node and the atria so both the P waves and QRS complexes are absent. SA block can be an isolated event or can occur frequently.

First Degree SA Block

The delay of the SA node's impulse from reaching the atria is unable to be recorded on an ECG.

Second Degree SA Block Wenckebach

It is due to the progressive difficulty of the depolarization wave in reaching the atria until finally it is unable to do so. It is characterized by a P-P cycle that gets progressively shorter until a ventricular pause occurs. The pause measures less than twice the preceding P-P cycle. There are no P waves or QRS complexes during the pause.

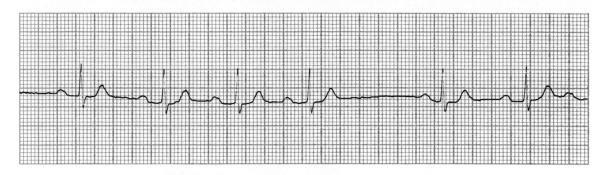

Sinus rhythm with first degree AV block and second degree SA block Wenckebach.

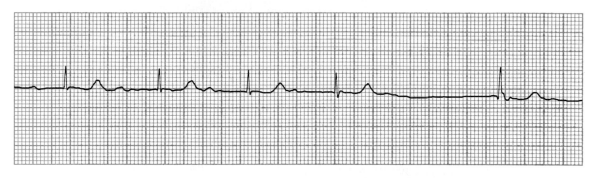

Sinus rhythm with first degree AV block and second degree SA block Wenckebach. The pause is terminated by a junctional escape beat.

SA Block Mobitz

SA block Mobitz is an intermittent blockage of the sinus node's impulses from reaching and depolarizing the atria. This is characterized by a constant P-P cycle before the ventricular pause. The ventricular pause contains no P waves or QRS complexes and measures 2, 3, or more times the length of the P-P cycle which represents the inability of the SA node's impulse to reach the atria once, twice, or more times. If more than one P wave in a row is blocked junctional and ventricular escape beats usually terminate the pause.

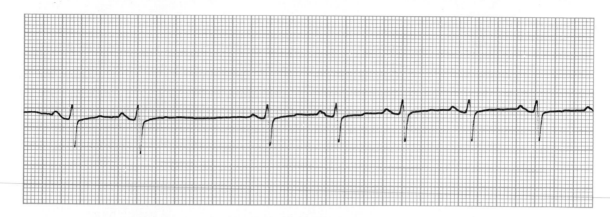

Sinus rhythm with intermittent 2:1 second degree SA block Mobitz.

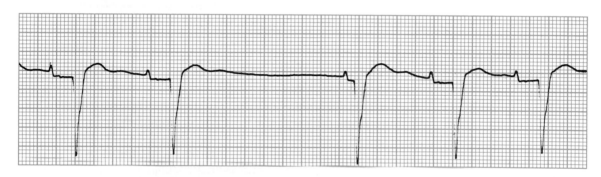

Sinus bradycardia with bundle branch block, first degree AV block, and second degree SA block Mobitz. The pause is terminated by a junctional escape beat.

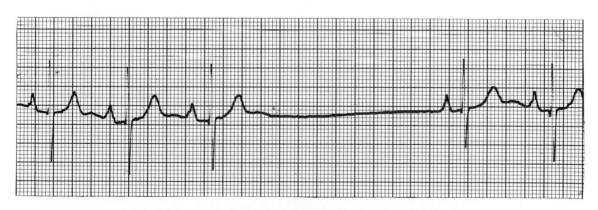

Sinus rhythm with first degree AV block and 3:1 second degree SA block Mobitz.

215

Differential Diagnosis

Second degree SA block Wenckebach and sinus arrhythmia are often indistinguishable from one another on an ECG. Both arrhythmias have P-P cycles which shorten and R-R cycles which lengthen. The only clue to identification is that sinus arrhythmia usually varies with respiration as the R-R cycles gradually shorten and then gradually lengthen. Second degree SA block Wenckebach shows a gradual shortening of the P-P cycle but an abrupt lengthening. Although sinus arrhythmia can display this abrupt lengthening, it is not as common an occurrence except in young children.

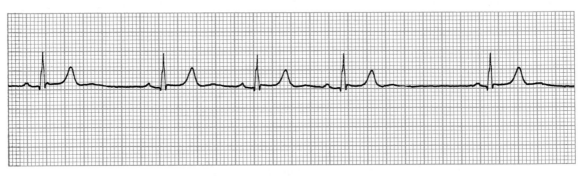

This strip is typical of sinus arrhythmia as the heart rate waxes and wanes with respiration. Although the P-P cycle shortens before the pause and the pause is less than twice the preceding P-P cycle, an overall assessment of the strip favors sinus arrhythmia over SA block Wenckebach.

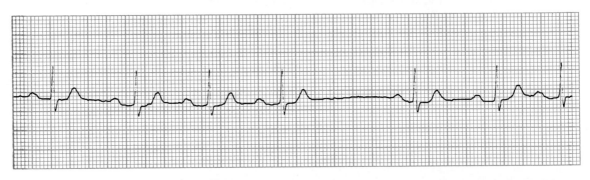

The abruptness of the ventricular pause is not generally typical of sinus arrhythmia except in young children. The shortening P-P cycle before the pause confirms SA block Wenckebach.

The ventricular pauses demonstrated in both second degree SA block Wenckebach and Mobitz can be confused with the pause following a nonconducted APC. If an ectopic P wave can't be found in the previous T wave then SA block or sinus arrhythmia are the other options for diagnosis.

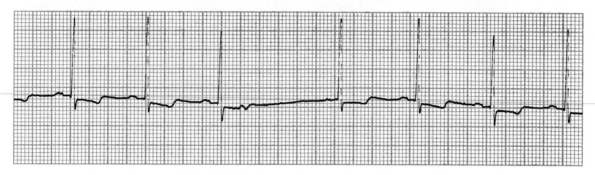

Sinus rhythm with a nonconducted APC. The ectopic P wave is clearly visible buried in the previous T wave ruling out the diagnosis of SA block.

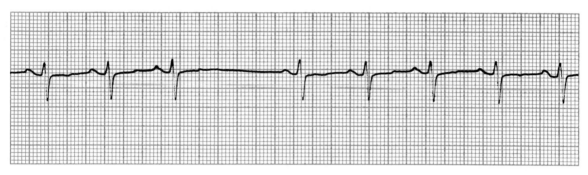

Sinus rhythm with 2:1 second degree SA block Mobitz. No ectopic P wave is visible in the T wave before the ventricular pause, ruling out the diagnosis of nonconducted APC.

PRACTICE ECGs

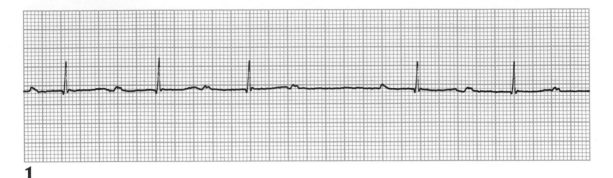

1

2

3

DIFFERENTIAL DIAGNOSIS OF ARRHYTHMIAS

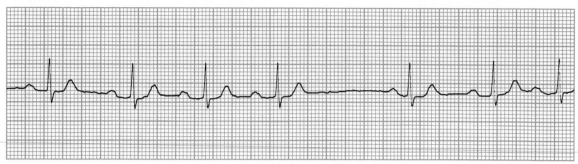

4

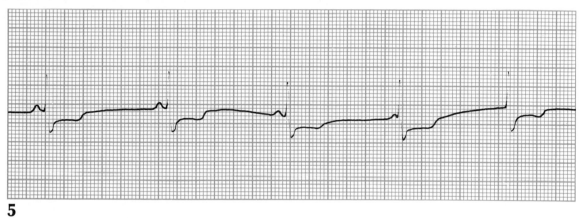

5

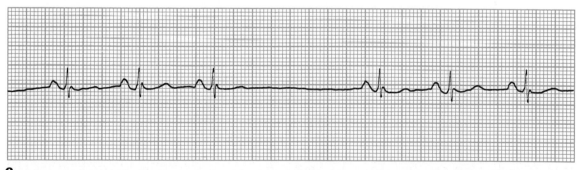

6

PRACTICE ECGs

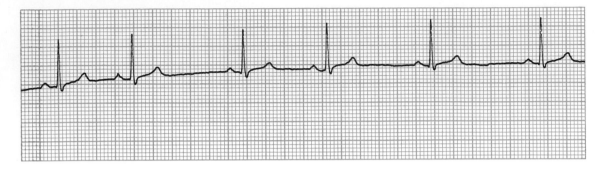

7

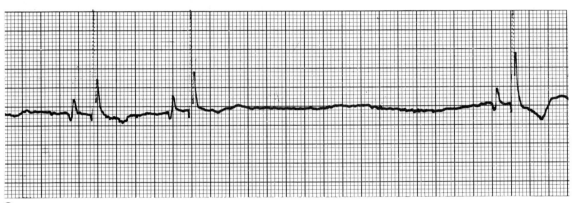

8

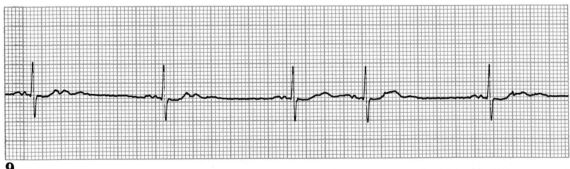

9

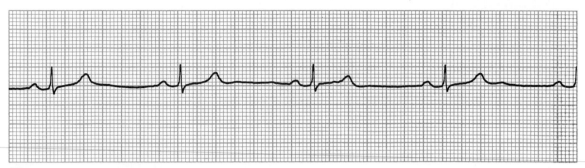

10

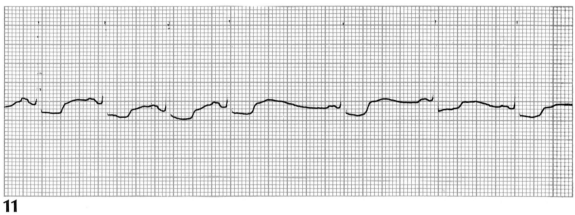

11

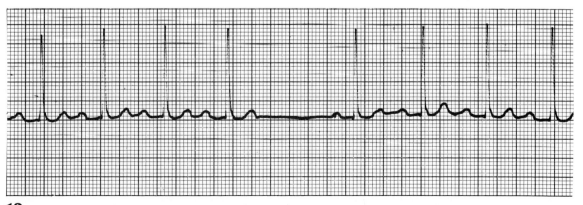

12

PRACTICE ECGs

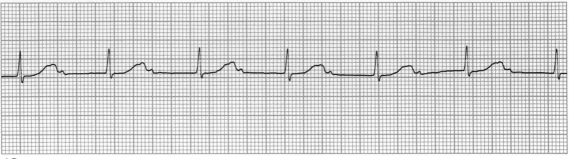

13

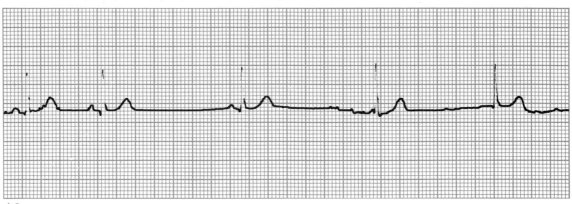

14

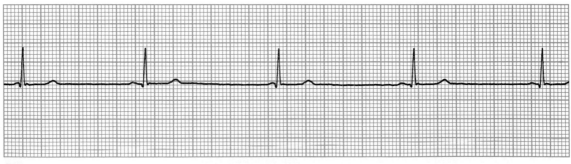

15

Practice ECG Answers

1. Sinus rhythm with first degree AV block and second degree AV block Wenckebach
2. Sinus rhythm with 2:1 second degree SA block Mobitz
3. Sinus rhythm with nonconducted APC
4. Sinus rhythm with first degree AV block and second degree SA block Wenckebach
5. Sinus arrhythmia with AV dissociation and a junctional escape rhythm
6. Sinus rhythm with 2:1 second degree SA block Mobitz
7. Sinus arrhythmia
8. Sinus bradycardia with first degree AV block and 3:1 second degree SA block Mobitz
9. Sinus rhythm with four nonconducted APCs
10. Sinus bradycardia
11. Sinus rhythm with second degree SA block Wenckebach
12. Sinus rhythm with a nonconducted APC
13. Sinus rhythm with marked first degree AV block
14. Sinus rhythm with 2:1 second degree SA block Mobitz with two junctional escape beats
15. Sinus bradycardia with AV dissociation and a junctional escape rhythm

10

WPW

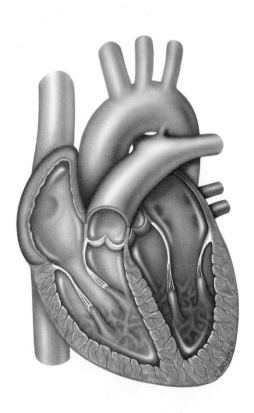

WPW

WPW

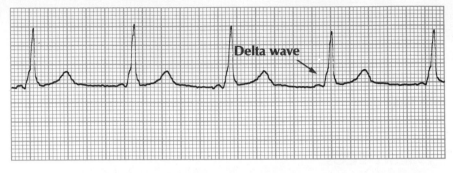

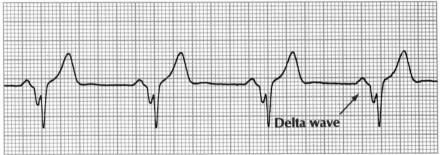

CRITERIA

1. A shortened PR interval is present in sinus rhythm

2. A delta wave is present

3. There are variations in QRS width and configuration

4. Supraventricular tachycardias are prone to occur

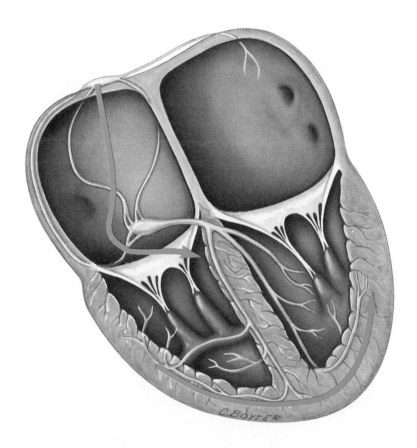

WPW is the rapid conduction of supraventricular impulses to the ventricles through an accessory pathway between the atria and ventricles which bypasses the AV node. During sinus rhythm, it is characterized by a shortened PR interval, which represents the shortened conduction time from atria to ventricles, and a wide and bizarre QRS complex with a **delta wave**. The delta wave is the slurring of the initial portion of the QRS complex. This distortion of the QRS complex occurs as one ventricle depolarizes first as it receives the electrical stimulation via the accessory pathway, and the other ventricle depolarizes with delay as it is depolarized abnormally through connections in the ventricular myocardium. The sinus impulses conduct to the ventricles simultaneously through both the accessory pathway and through normal AV conduction pathways. There can be degrees of variation in the shape and width of the QRS depending on the amount of ventricular myocardium depolarized normally and the amount occurring through the accessory pathway.

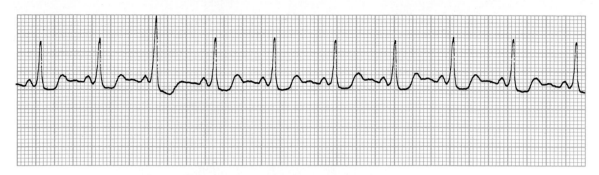

Sinus rhythm with WPW. The third beat displays a variation in the QRS complex as more of the ventricular myocardium is depolarized through the accessory pathway.

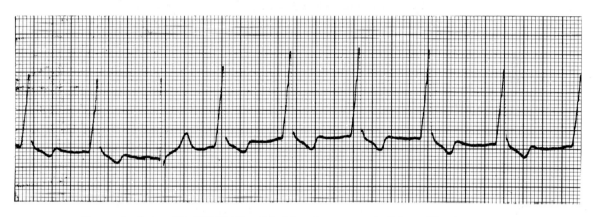

Sinus rhythm with WPW. The third beat represents intermittent depolarization through normal conduction pathways. The other complexes display shortened PR intervals, delta waves, and widened QRS complexes.

Supraventricular tachycardias tend to occur frequently and the wide and bizarre QRS complexes accompanying the rapid rates make the distinction between ventricular tachycardia and supraventricular tachycardia with WPW difficult.

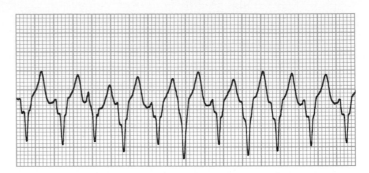

Atrial fibrillation with WPW. The irregular ventricular response leads to the diagnosis of atrial fibrillation and the widened QRS and presence of a negative delta wave leads to the diagnosis of WPW.

Differential Diagnosis

WPW produces wide and bizarre QRS complexes and presents the same interpretation problems as does aberration. The biggest dilemmas are the supraventricular tachycardias mimicking ventricular tachycardias. Look for irregular R-R cycles which would indicate atrial fibrillation, or look for ectopic P waves preceding or following the QRS complexes which would confirm supraventricular tachycardia.

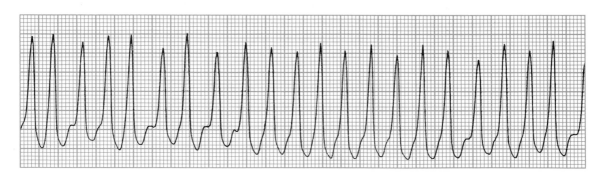

Atrial fibrillation with WPW.

DIFFERENTIAL DIAGNOSIS OF ARRHYTHMIAS

WPW displays a shortened PR interval which could be mistaken for the sinus P wave floating into the QRS complex during AV dissociation. But during AV dissociation the sinus P wave will float into and out of the QRS complex producing a varying PR interval. The PR interval in WPW will be short but will remain constant.

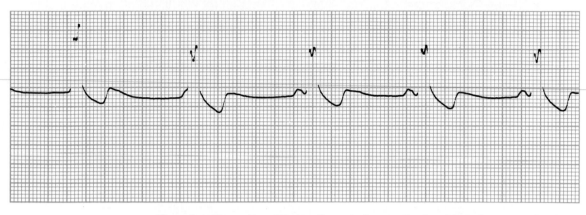

Sinus bradycardia with AV dissociation and a junctional escape rhythm with bundle branch block. The varying PR interval rules out WPW.

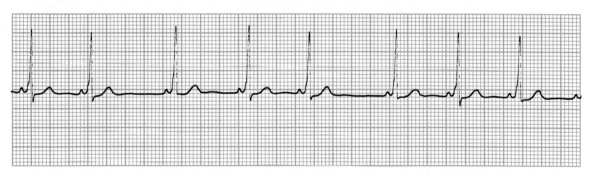

Sinus arrhythmia with WPW. The constant PR interval rules out AV dissociation. Note the slight variation in the QRS configuration.

PRACTICE ECGs

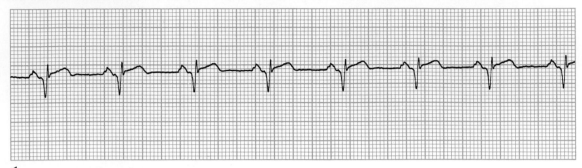

1

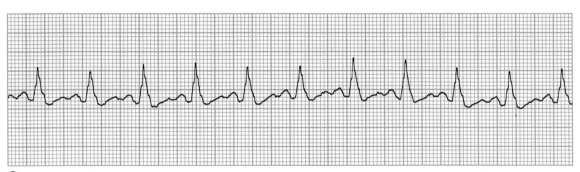

2

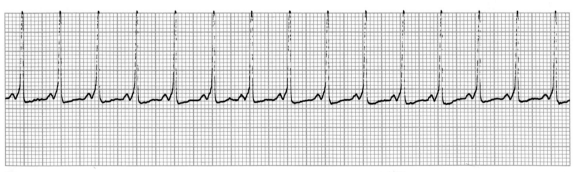

3

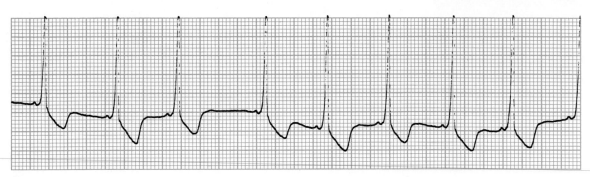

4

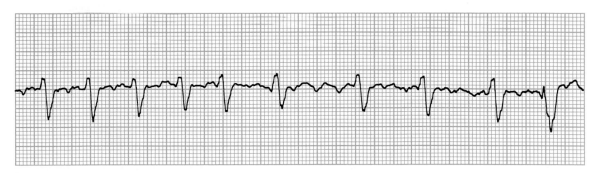

5

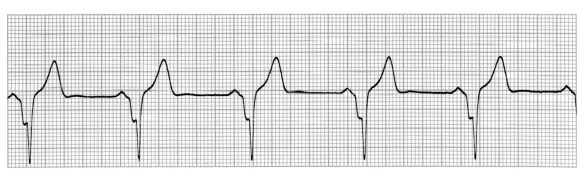

6

PRACTICE ECGs

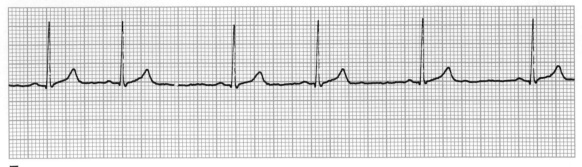

7

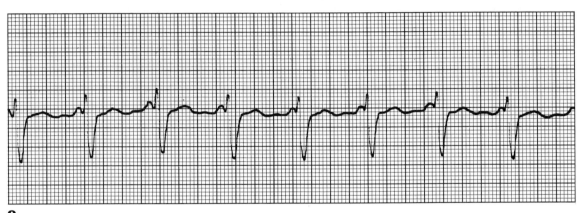

8

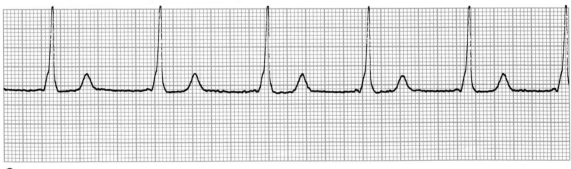

9

DIFFERENTIAL DIAGNOSIS OF ARRHYTHMIAS

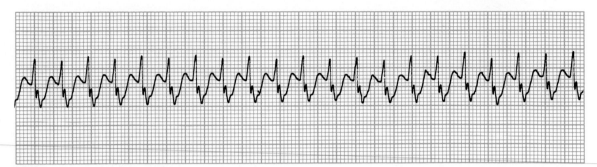

10

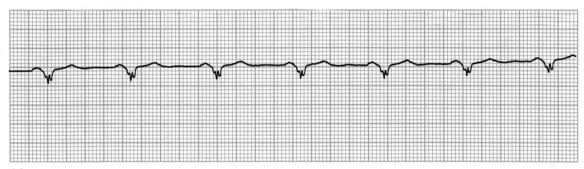

11

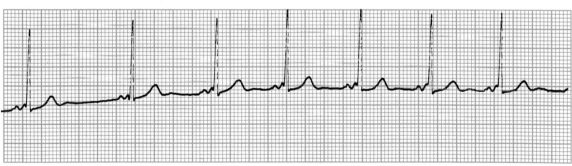

12

PRACTICE ECGs

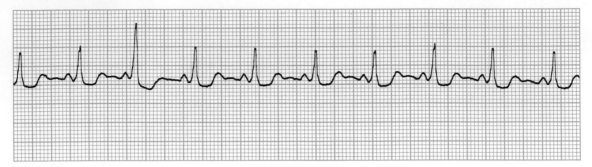

13

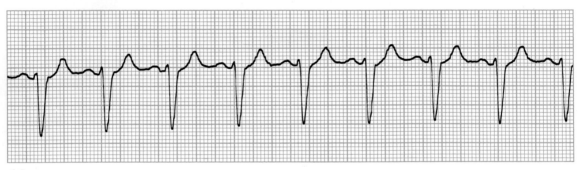

14

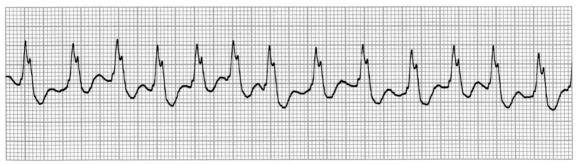

15

DIFFERENTIAL DIAGNOSIS OF ARRHYTHMIAS

Practice ECG Answers

1. Sinus rhythm with WPW
2. Sinus tachycardia with bundle branch block
3. Sinus tachycardia with WPW
4. Sinus arrhythmia with WPW
5. Atrial fibrillation with bundle branch block
6. Sinus bradycardia with WPW
7. Sinus arrhythmia
8. Sinus rhythm with AV dissociation and an accelerated junctional rhythm with bundle branch block versus an accelerated ventricular rhythm
9. Sinus bradycardia with WPW
10. Supraventricular tachycardia with aberration versus ventricular tachycardia
11. Sinus rhythm with WPW
12. Sinus arrhythmia with WPW
13. Sinus rhythm with WPW
14. Sinus rhythm with bundle branch block
15. Atrial fibrillation with bundle branch block

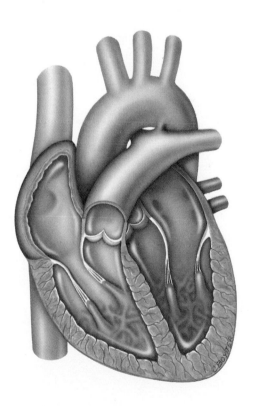

11

REVIEW ECGs

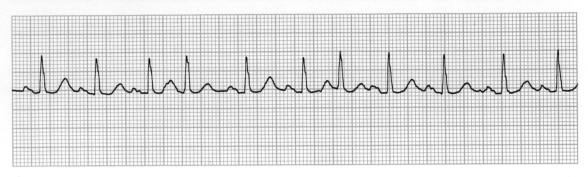

1

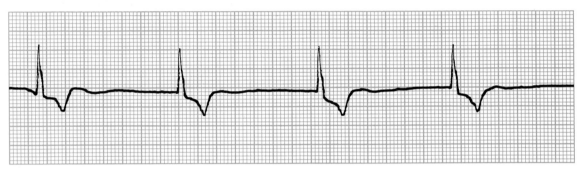

2

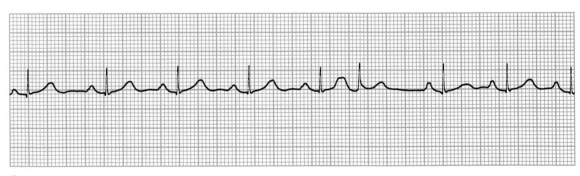

3

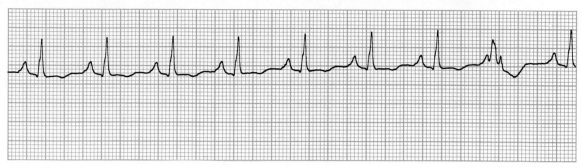

4

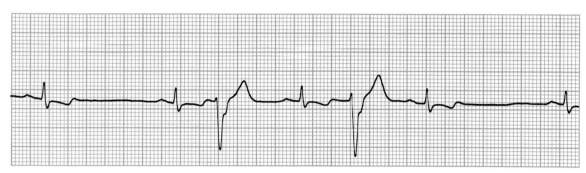

5

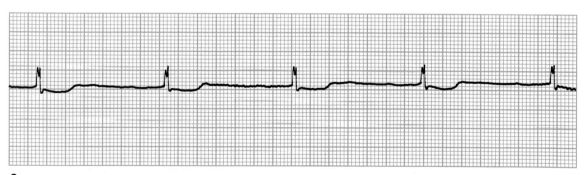

6

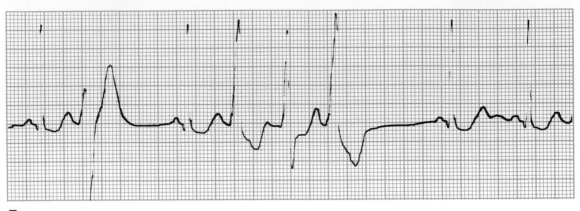

7

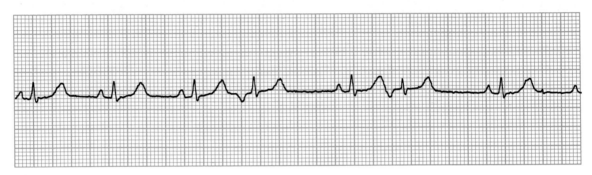

8

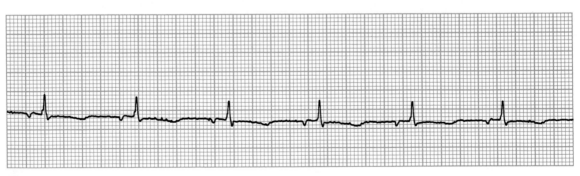

9

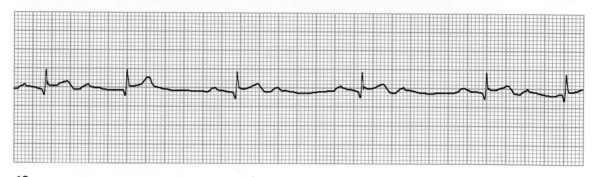

10

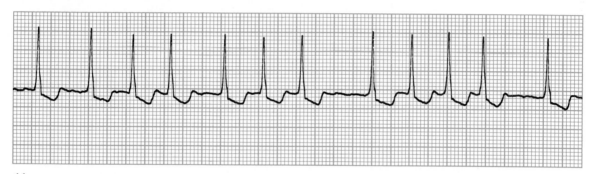

11

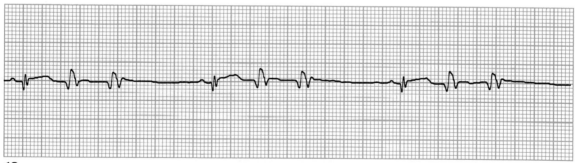

12

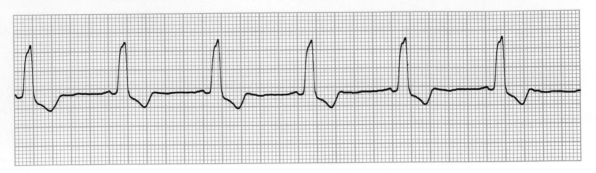

13

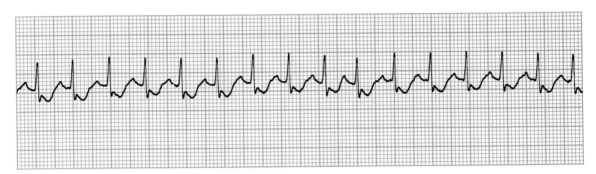

14

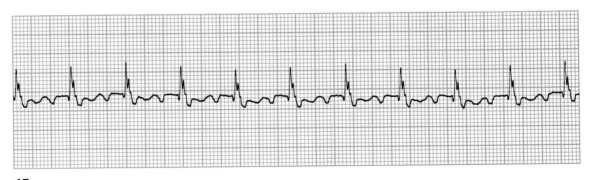

15

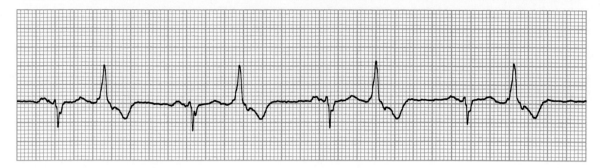

16

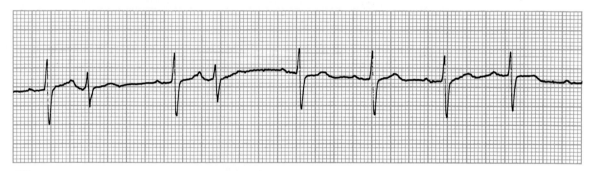

17

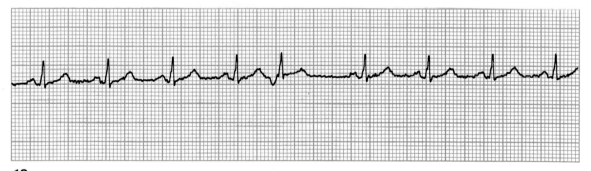

18

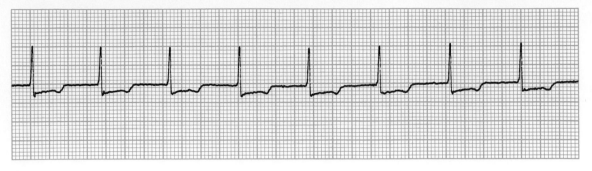

19

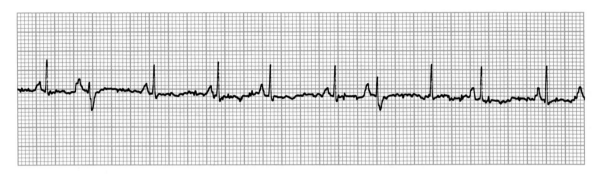

20

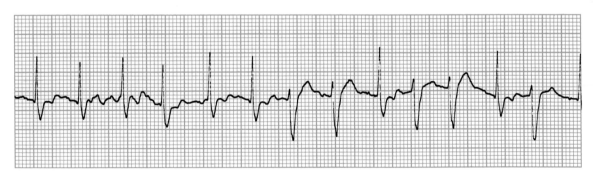

21

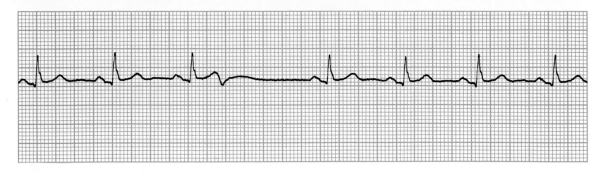

22

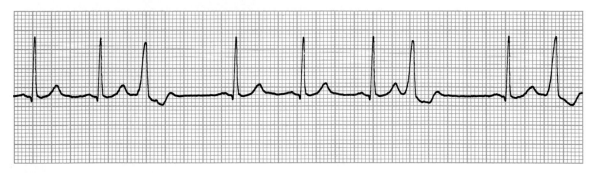

23

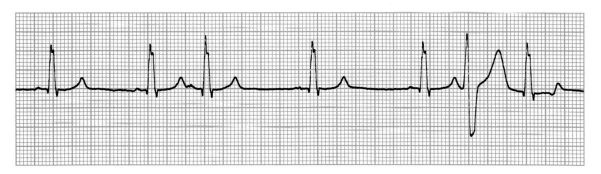

24

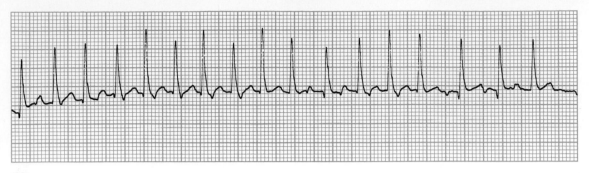

25

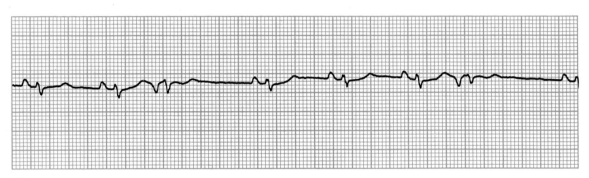

26

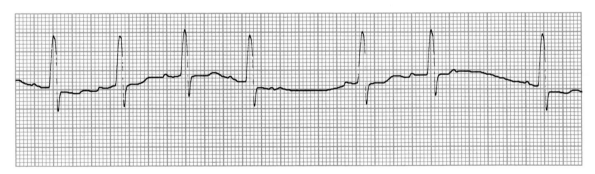

27

DIFFERENTIAL DIAGNOSIS OF ARRHYTHMIAS

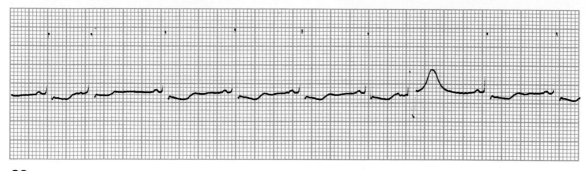

28

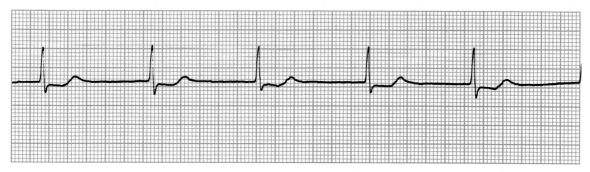

29

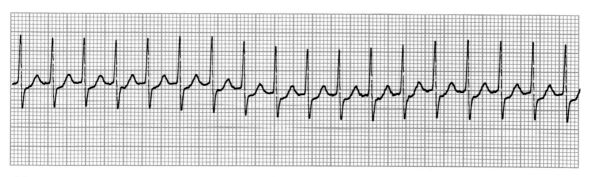

30

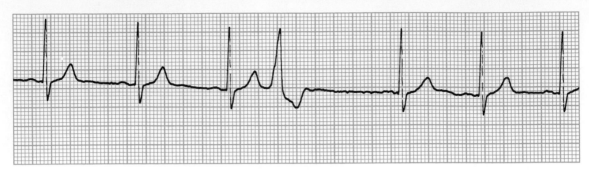

31

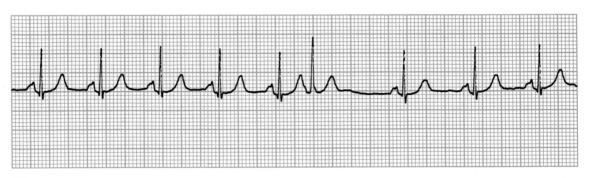

32

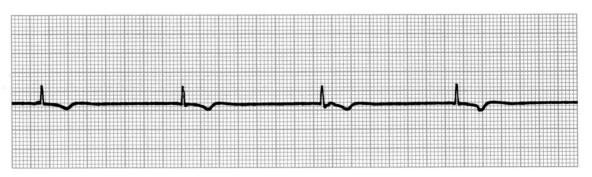

33

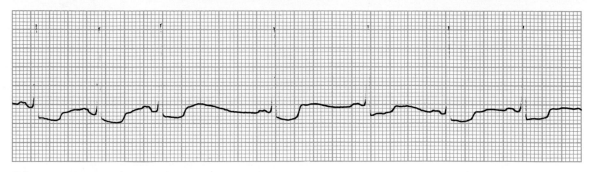

34

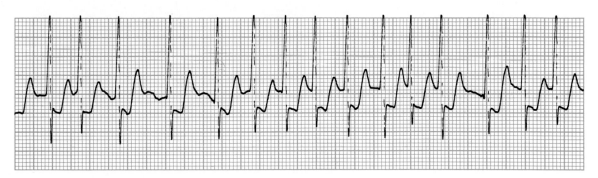

35

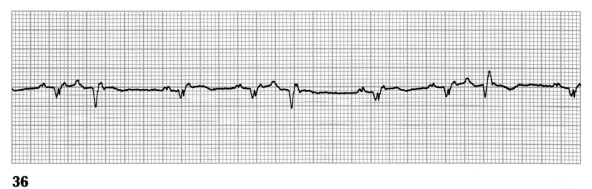

36

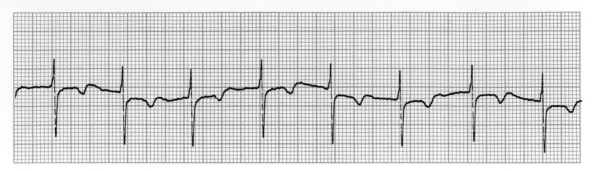

37

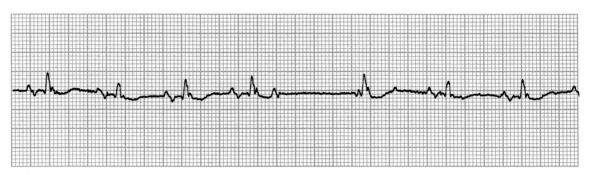

38

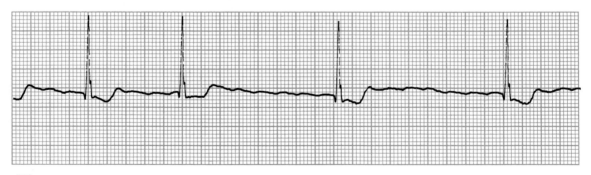

39

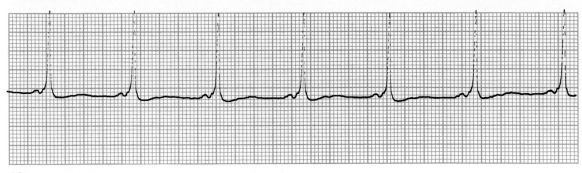

40

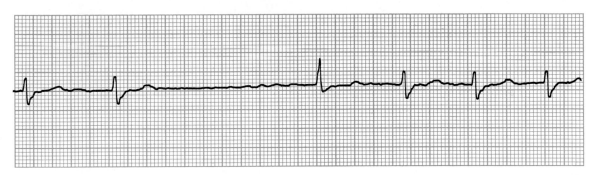

41

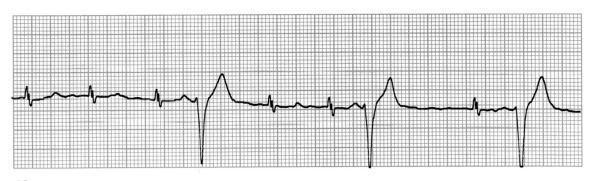

42

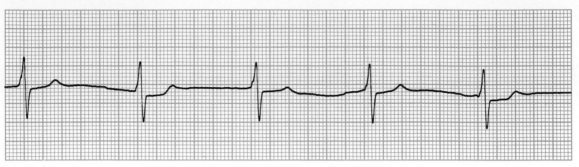

43

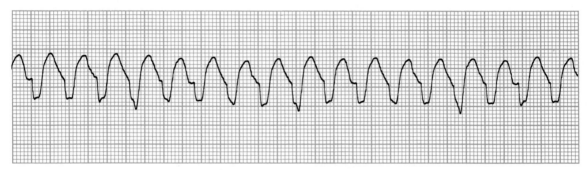

44

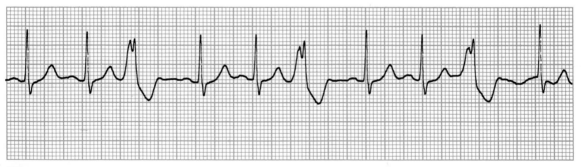

45

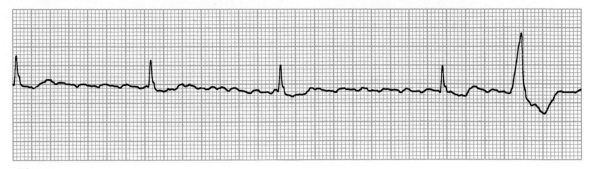

46

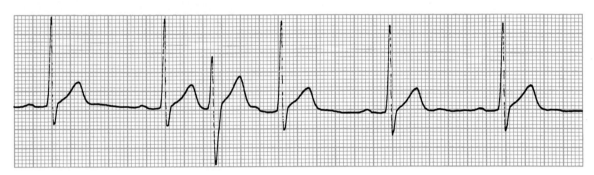

47

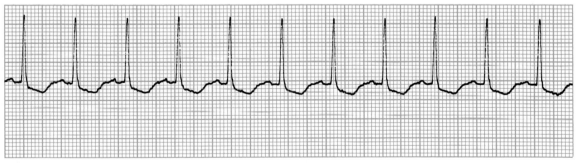

48

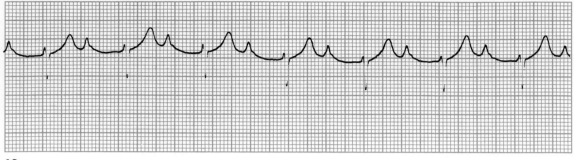

49

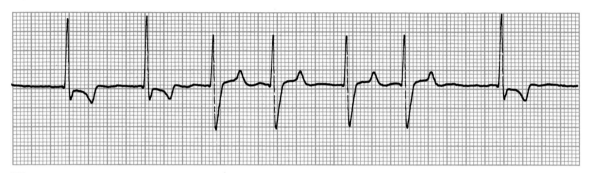

50

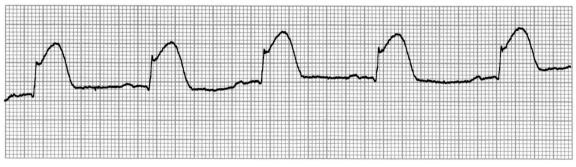

51

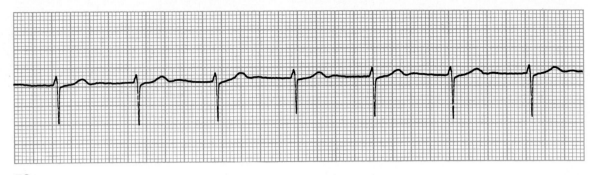

52

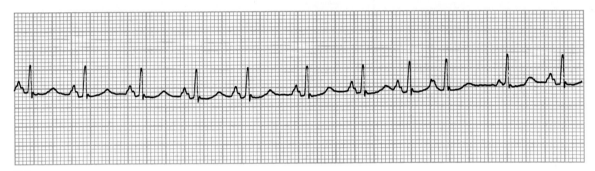

53

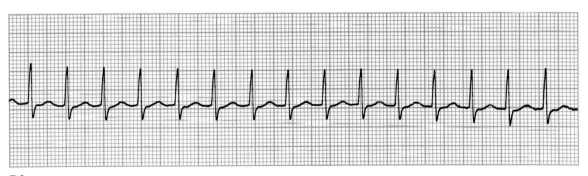

54

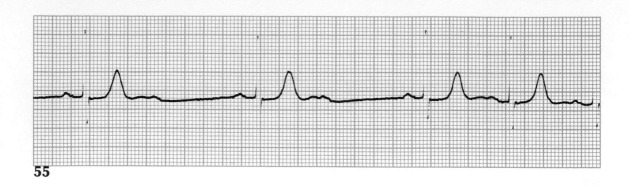

55

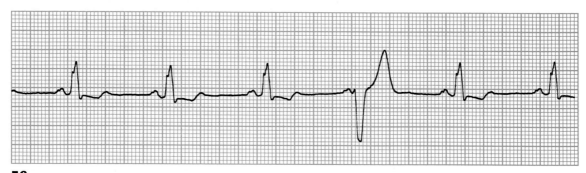

56

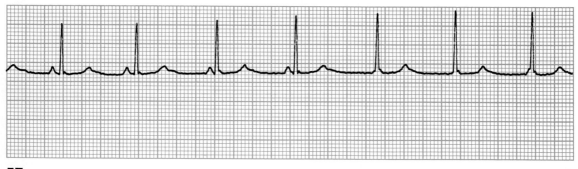

57

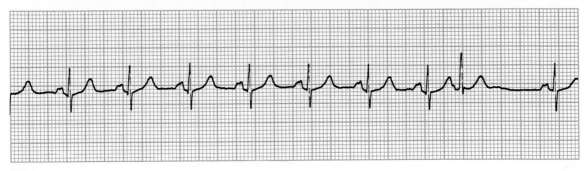

58

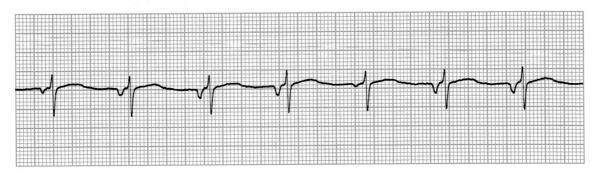

59

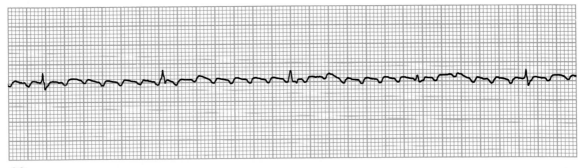

60

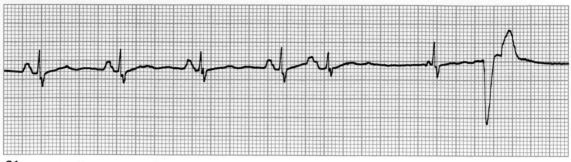

61

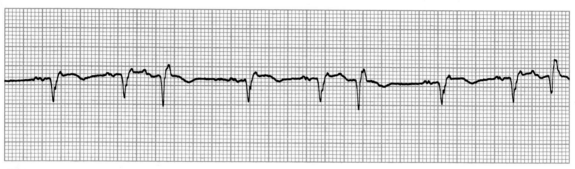

62

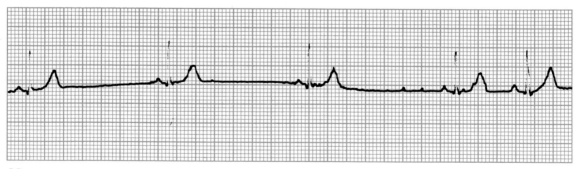

63

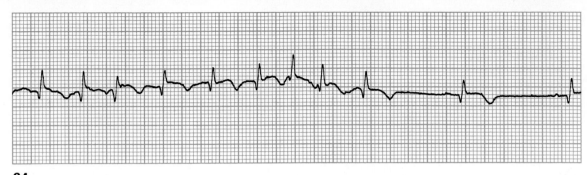

64

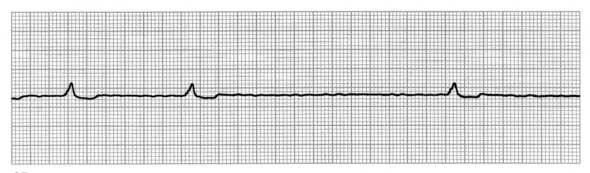

65

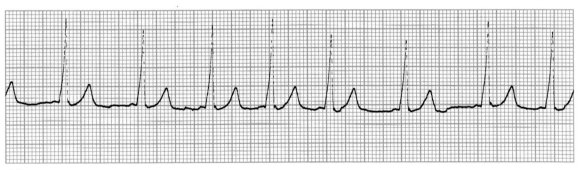

66

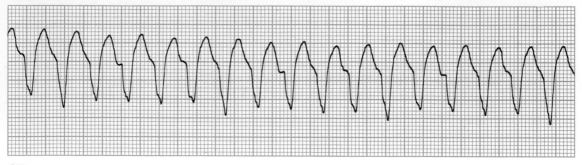

67

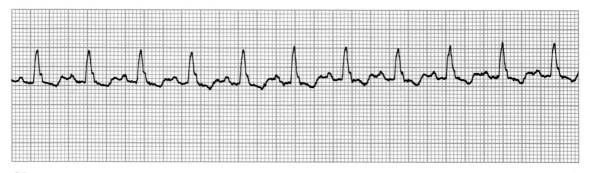

68

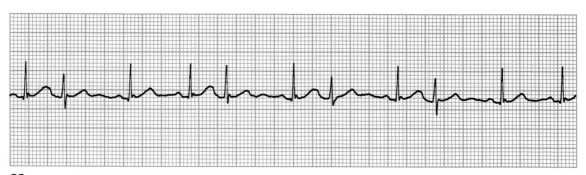

69

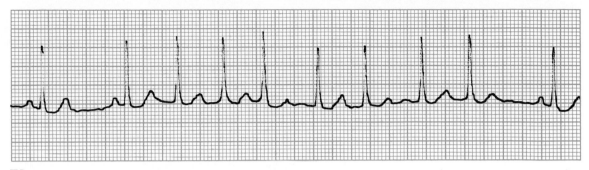

70

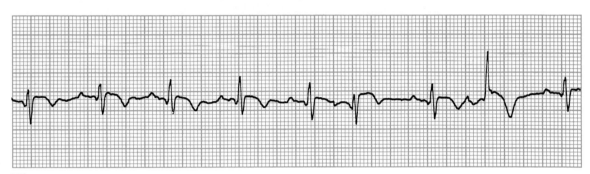

71

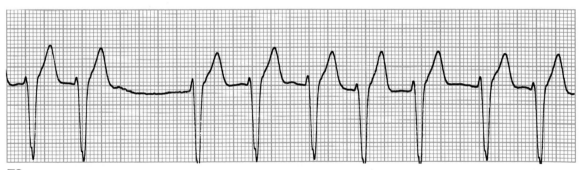

72

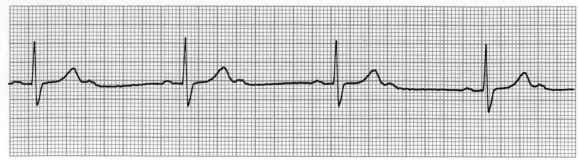

73

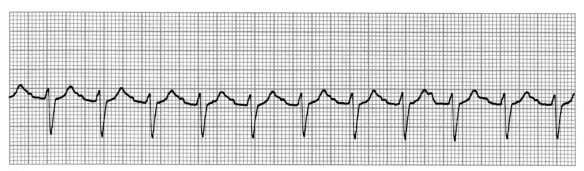

74

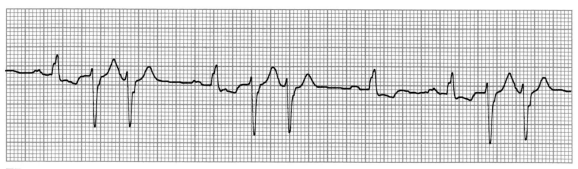

75

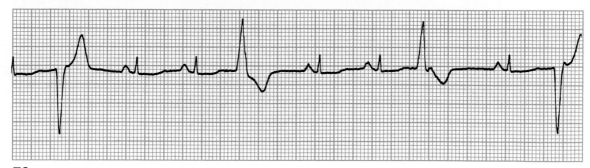

76

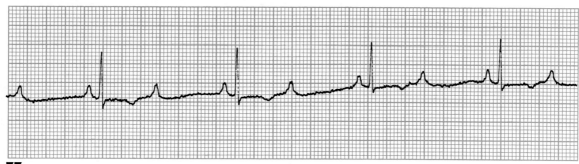

77

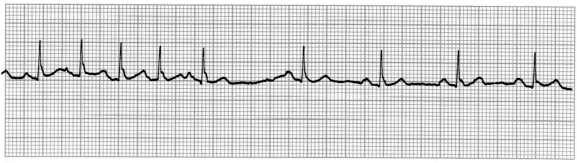

78

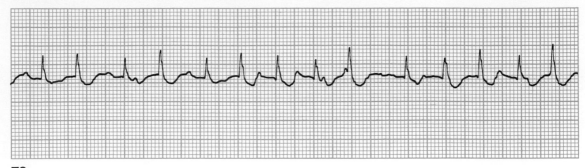

79

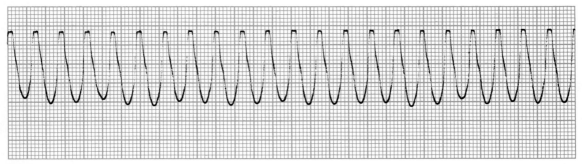

80

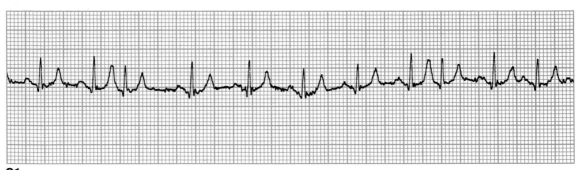

81

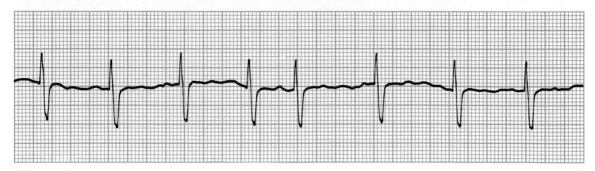

82

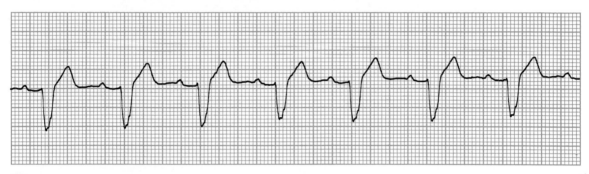

83

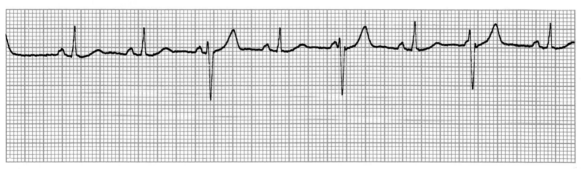

84

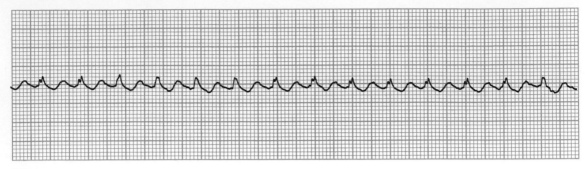

85

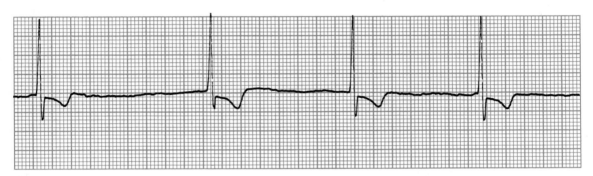

86

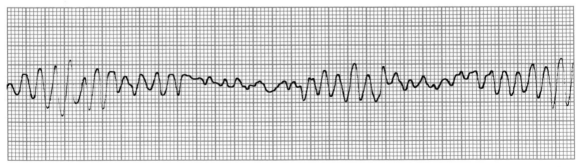

87

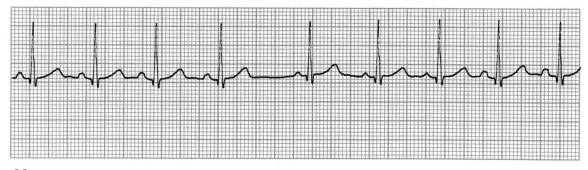

88

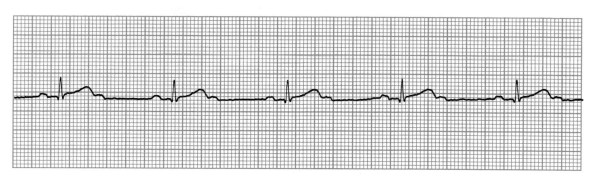

89

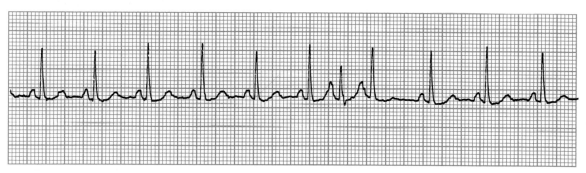

90

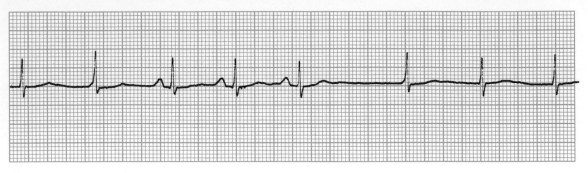

91

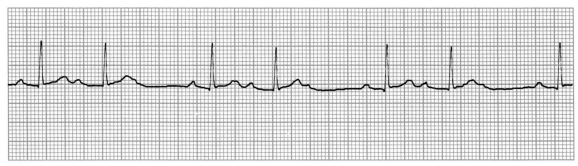

92

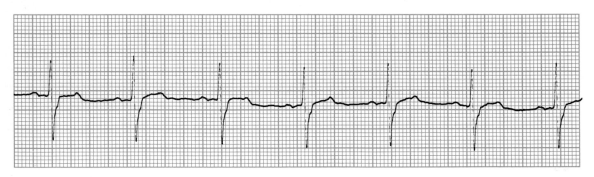

93

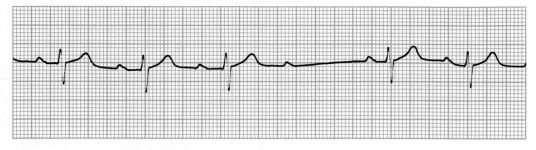

94

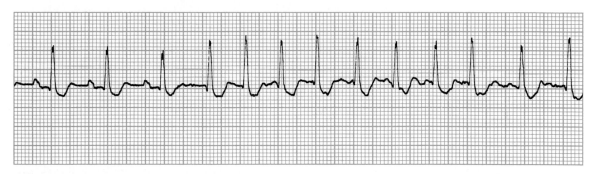

95

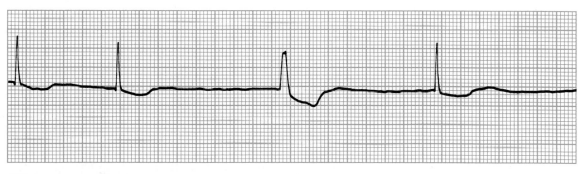

96

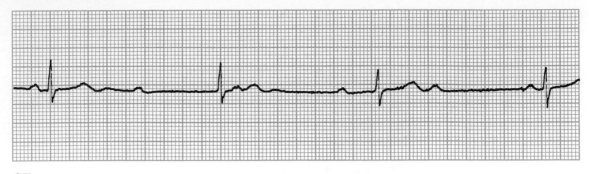

97

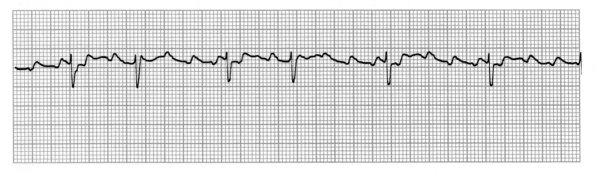

98

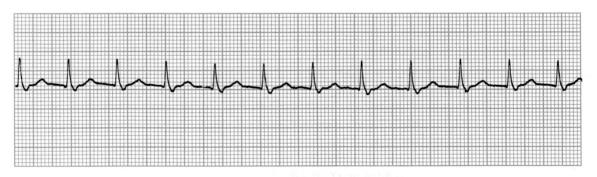

99

Answers to Review ECGs

1. Sinus tachycardia with two isolated atrial premature contractions
2. Junctional escape rhythm
3. Sinus rhythm with one isolated atrial premature contraction
4. Sinus rhythm with one end diastolic ventricular premature contraction
5. Sinus bradycardia with two unifocal interpolated ventricular premature contractions
6. Junctional escape rhythm
7. Sinus rhythm with one isolated VPC and three multifocal ventricular premature contractions in a row
8. Sinus rhythm with two isolated junctional premature contractions
9. Accelerated junctional rhythm
10. Sinus rhythm with first degree and second degree AV block Wenckebach
11. Atrial fibrillation
12. Sinus rhythm with pairs of unifocal ventricular premature beats in bigeminy
13. Sinus rhythm with bundle branch block
14. Atrial tachycardia
15. Paroxysmal atrial tachycardia with 2:1 block
16. Sinus rhythm with four unifocal ventricular premature beats in bigeminy
17. Sinus rhythm with two atrial premature contractions with aberration
18. Sinus rhythm with one isolated junctional premature contraction
19. Accelerated junctional rhythm
20. Sinus rhythm with four isolated atrial premature contractions, two with aberration
21. Atrial fibrillation with aberrant beats
22. Sinus rhythm with one nonconducted atrial premature contraction
23. Sinus rhythm with three isolated unifocal ventricular premature contractions
24. Sinus bradycardia with bundle branch block, one isolated atrial premature contraction and one interpolated ventricular premature contraction
25. Multifocal atrial tachycardia
26. Sinus rhythm with two isolated junctional premature contractions
27. Sinus rhythm with bundle branch block and two nonconducted atrial premature contractions
28. Sinus rhythm with two isolated atrial premature contractions—one with aberration
29. Junctional escape rhythm
30. Supraventricular tachycardia
31. Sinus rhythm with one isolated ventricular premature contraction
32. Sinus rhythm with one isolated atrial premature contraction with aberrancy

33. Junctional escape rhythm
34. Sinus rhythm with second degree SA block Wenckebach
35. Atrial fibrillation
36. Sinus rhythm with three isolated atrial premature contractions with varying degrees of aberration
37. Accelerated junctional rhythm
38. Sinus rhythm with bundle branch block, first degree AV block, and one nonconducted atrial premature contraction followed by a junctional escape beat
39. Atrial fibrillation with high grade AV block
40. Sinus rhythm with WPW
41. Atrial fibrillation with bundle branch block and a long ventricular pause terminated by a ventricular escape beat
42. Atrial fibrillation with three, isolated unifocal ventricular premature contractions
43. Junctional escape rhythm
44. Ventricular tachycardia
45. Sinus tachycardia with three isolated, unifocal ventricular premature contractions in trigeminy
46. Atrial fibrillation with high grade AV block and one isolated ventricular premature contraction
47. Sinus bradycardia with first degree AV block and one interpolated ventricular premature contraction
48. Sinus tachycardia
49. Sinus rhythm with first degree AV block
50. Atrial fibrillation with four aberrant beats
51. Sinus bradycardia with first degree AV block and marked ST elevation
52. Accelerated junctional rhythm
53. Sinus tachycardia with one isolated atrial premature contraction followed by a junctional escape beat
54. Junctional tachycardia
55. Sinus rhythm with first degree and second degree AV block Mobitz
56. Sinus rhythm with bundle branch block and one end diastolic ventricular premature contraction
57. AV dissociation between sinus rhythm and an accelerated junctional rhythm
58. Sinus rhythm with one isolated atrial premature contraction with aberration
59. Accelerated junctional rhythm
60. Atrial flutter with high grade AV block
61. Sinus rhythm with one isolated atrial premature contraction followed by a junctional escape beat and a ventricular premature contraction
62. Sinus rhythm with three isolated atrial premature contractions in trigeminy with varying degrees of aberration
63. Sinus rhythm with second degree SA block Mobitz

DIFFERENTIAL DIAGNOSIS OF ARRHYTHMIAS

64. Atrial fibrillation followed by sinus bradycardia
65. Atrial fibrillation with high grade AV block
66. Sinus arrhythmia and WPW
67. Ventricular tachycardia
68. Sinus tachycardia with bundle branch block
69. Sinus rhythm with four isolated atrial premature contractions with varying degrees of aberration
70. Sinus rhythm followed by a burst of atrial fibrillation and reverting back to sinus rhythm
71. Sinus rhythm with two isolated atrial premature contractions, one with aberration
72. Atrial fibrillation with bundle branch block
73. Sinus arrhythmia with first degree and second degree AV block Mobitz
74. Sinus tachycardia with first degree AV block
75. Sinus rhythm with first degree AV block with unifocal ventricular premature contractions in pairs
76. Sinus rhythm with four isolated multifocal ventricular premature contractions
77. Sinus rhythm with second degree AV block Mobitz
78. Atrial tachycardia reverting to sinus rhythm
79. Multifocal atrial tachycardia
80. Ventricular flutter
81. Sinus tachycardia with two isolated atrial premature contractions
82. Sinus rhythm with bundle branch block and one isolated atrial premature contraction
83. Sinus rhythm with bundle branch block and first degree AV block
84. Sinus rhythm with three unifocal end diastolic ventricular premature contractions
85. Atrial flutter with 2:1 block
86. Atrial fibrillation with high grade AV block
87. Ventricular fibrillation
88. Sinus arrhythmia
89. Sinus rhythm with first degree and second degree AV block Mobitz
90. Sinus tachycardia with a pair of atrial premature contractions, the first displaying aberration
91. AV dissociation between sinus rhythm and an accelerated junctional rhythm
92. Sinus rhythm with first degree and second degree AV block Wenckebach
93. Paroxysmal atrial tachycardia with 2:1 AV block
94. Sinus rhythm with first degree AV block and second degree AV block Wenckebach
95. Sinus tachycardia reverting to atrial fibrillation
96. Atrial fibrillation with one ventricular escape beat

97. Complete AV block with sinus bradycardia and a junctional escape rhythm
98. Atrial flutter with varying block
99. Junctional tachycardia